THE STROKE RECOVERY BOOK

KIP BURKMAN, M.D.

Addicus Books, Inc.
Omaha, Nebraska

An Addicus Nonfiction Book

ISBN 1-886039-30-5

Cover design by Jeff Reiner
Illustrations by Bob Hogenmiller
Photos by David Jenkins / Shelton Hendricks, model
Typography by Linda Dageforde

This book is not intended to substitute for a physician, nor does the author intend to give medical advice contrary to that of an attending physician.

Library of Congress Cataloging-in-Publication Data

Burkman, Kip, 1953-
    The stroke recovery book : a guide for patients and families / by Kip Burkman.
      p. cm.
    Includes index.
    ISBN 1-886039-30-5
    1. Cerebrovascular disease—Popular works.   I. Title
RC388.5.B87 1998   98-6547
616.8'1—dc21   CIP

Addicus Books, Inc.

P.O. Box 45327
Omaha, Nebraska 68145
Web site: http://members.aol.com/addicusbks

Printed in the United States of America
10 9 8 7 6 5 4 3 2 1

To my wife, Christine and my mother, Bettelou.
Through their love I have learned my most important lessons.

Contents

Part I - Anatomy of a Stroke

   A "brain attack," warning signs of stroke, major causes of strokes, brain anatomy, types of strokes, stroke deficits

Part II - Impairments and Complications Caused by Stroke

   Perception, vision, visual field cuts, double-vision, touch, limb numbness, intellect, behavior, emotions, anger, depression
   Aphasia, dysarthria, speech therapy evaluation, accessory communication
   Apraxia and neglect, recovering muscle strength, regaining coordination, how long will it take?

Part III - Recovery and Rehabilitation

Part IV - Preventing Strokes

Acknowledgments

A number of individuals played a role in the development of this book. I am grateful to them all. I express deep gratitude to patients and families who, through the years, have helped me learn the art of medicine. Through these people, I have seen the strength of the human spirit in the face of life-changing obstacles.

I wish to thank my colleagues at the Immanuel Medical Center who continually help me understand the science of medicine. I also thank the many other health professionals and therapists who shared their perspectives for this book. I especially thank Julie Pribyl, Julie Meyer, Sharon Woodard, and Sister Patricia Mokler for their encouragement during the time I was writing the manuscript.

Finally, I thank Rod Colvin of Addicus Books for his support and for asking me to write this book.

Introduction

As a rehabilitation physician, I have treated hundreds of stroke patients over the last fourteen years. I have seen patients and families being swept into a tailspin of confusion and overpowering emotion as the result of stroke. One of the biggest fears, for both patients and families, is the fear of the unknown. What to expect? What happens next?

My goal in writing this book is to provide answers to some of your questions so that you'll be better prepared to navigate your way though this stressful time. Remember, every patient is different, so it's not possible to cover specific issues here. Instead, I've tried to provide a basic knowledge of strokes within these pages.

If you are a family member or friend to someone who has had a stroke, I would advise that you first educate yourself about stroke and rehabilitation. Secondly, I suggest that communicate with your loved one's caregivers. Effective communication can go a long way toward reducing your anxiety. And, patients, who have supportive families and friends, have better recovery outcomes. As much as possible, get involved in the recovery and rehabilitation.

Remember also, when suddenly afflicted by a devastating illness, patients often withdraw mentally and emotionally as a way to cope. Unfortunately then, the patient doesn't always hear or understand what he or she is being told—all the more reason for families to be informed and participating. So my final word of advice: be patient and supportive with the stroke patient in your life.

Although the world is full of suffering,
it is full also of overcoming it.

Helen Keller
1880-1968

Part I

Anatomy of a Stroke

1

What Is a Stroke?

Imagine, for a moment, you're looking at familiar surroundings but nothing you see makes sense. The world looks as if it's been cut in half. You have a pounding headache. Suddenly, you're aware of a spreading warmth between your legs. You've wet your pants. You've also fallen to the floor. No matter how hard you struggle to get up, you can't. Neither your arm nor your leg will move. You try calling for help, but the words coming out of your mouth are gibberish. If you're alone, a frightening thought overwhelms you: *What if no one finds me?*

This scenario describes what it might be like if you suffer a stroke. A frightening proposition, indeed, especially in those first hours and days. You wonder if you will live. Will you be impaired? How long will rehabilitation take? How complete will recovery be? These are just a few of the questions that might race through your mind and those of new stroke patients and their loved ones. Unfortunately, there are no standard answers to these questions. However, for most individuals, the ability to understand and adapt to this new reality depends largely on the attitudes and efforts of family, friends, health-care professionals, and caregivers. This book contains basic information to help you understand the complexities of stroke and recovery so that the patient in your life may receive the best possible care and support.

Warning Signs of a Stroke

The symptoms of a stroke—too often ignored—may lead to damaging consequences.

- sudden weakness or paralysis of the face or any limb
- sudden numbness of the face or any limb
- sudden problems with the ability to speak or understand speech
- sudden blindness in an eye
- sudden onset of dizziness or problems with balance
- sudden difficulty swallowing
- sudden difficulty walking or with coordination

Obtain immediate medical attention if any of these symptoms appear. Rapid treatment of a stroke may prevent functional impairment and even save your life.

A "Brain Attack"

A *stroke* is a "brain attack" in the same way a blockage of blood flow to the heart is a "heart attack." A stroke occurs when an area of the brain is deprived of blood flow. Most commonly, this happens when blood vessels are blocked by a clot or have become too narrow for blood to pass through. A stroke may also occur when a blood vessel bursts and leaks blood into the brain, causing damage. A lack of blood pumped to the brain, the result of a heart attack, may also cause a stroke.

When blood flow to the brain stops suddenly, a person will fall unconscious in about twelve seconds. Since the brain relies on the glucose and oxygen carried by blood cells for energy, brain cells will begin to die after about four minutes without these nutrients. This is a serious problem. Unlike other body tissues that have the ability to repair themselves over time, brain tissue is highly specialized and is less able to recover.

Major Causes of Stroke

Thrombosis

The leading cause of stroke is *thrombosis,* the gradual clogging of blood vessels with cholesterol or clotted blood. It is similar to the deposit of lime scale in water pipes. Eventually enough scale accumulates to narrow or totally shut off the flow of water. In blood vessels, a buildup of cholesterol from years of eating a high-fat diet may have the same effect. Progression toward a stroke may be either sudden or incremental. Symptoms and conditions may alternately worsen or improve over hours or weeks.

Embolism

Embolism, the second major cause of stroke, occurs when a clot formed in a blood vessel somewhere in the body breaks off, enters the brain's circulatory system, and travels until it encounters an artery it can't pass through. The *middle cerebral artery,* located in the middle portion of the brain, is most often affected by emboli. Clots may be caused by *platelets,* part of the blood's clotting mechanism, or by cholesterol in the neck arteries that softens and breaks off into a blood vessel. When a clot lodges in a blood vessel, the area of the brain served by that blood vessel may die. Sometimes clots break up into smaller pieces quickly enough to restore the blood flow. Some embolism patients experience a secondary problem: bleeding from damaged vessels where the emboli lodge.

> *My mother has changed in many ways from her stroke, but she is still the matriarch of our family. This bittersweet change has taught us to value every moment with her. I've learned to cherish the depth, beauty, and mystery of life.*
>
> *John*
> *Age 40*

5

The heart, as well as the neck, is a major source of clots. Clots from the heart can arise from abnormal heart rhythms, heart attacks, the placement of artificial heart valves, heart bypass operations, infections inside the heart, mitral valve prolapse (valves collapse inward, allowing blood to enter a chamber inappropriately) or damage to the heart valves from rheumatic heart disease. If a large clot that originates in the heart fragments, the brain may be showered with small pieces, causing multiple patterns of brain damage. These patterns often help a physician identify a stroke caused by emboli. A physician may perform a test, a *transthoracic* or *transesophageal echocardiogram,* to help determine whether an abnormality inside the heart is responsible for emboli. This procedure involves placing a special probe into the *esophagus,* the swallowing tube in the throat, and bouncing sound waves off the back of the heart to reveal pictures of the heart's structures and function, including clots inside the heart which may be responsible for the stroke.

After I had a stroke, I was worried about being able to earn a living. The stroke affected my right side so I'm learning to compensate with my left side. I will not stop trying to make progress.

Mary
Age 44

Hemorrhages

Hemorrhage is the third major cause of stroke. Hemorrhages can be caused by *aneurysms,* weakened blood vessels that form bubble-shaped projections and then break. A *subarachnoid hemorrhage* results from bleeding in the deeper cavities of the brain. An *intracerebral hemorrhage* occurs when a blood vessel bursts, leaking blood into the firm tissue of the brain. Pressure or blood vessel spasm from the bleeding can pinch surrounding blood vessels, shutting off more blood flow and producing further stroke effects.

Hemorrhagic strokes are the most deadly, due to the pressure they can produce on vital parts of the brain. Patients who survive bleeding strokes over thirty days often have fairly good functional outcomes. The most common cause of stroke by hemorrhage is poorly controlled high blood pressure, also known as *hypertension*. Other causes include malformations of blood vessels inside the brain, diseases of blood clotting, some types of liver disease, and brain tumors.

Hypotension

Hypotension, the fourth major cause of stroke, occurs when blood pressure falls to dangerously low levels. Not enough blood is pumped to the brain. The medical term for the resulting brain damage condition is *anoxic encephalopathy*. These patients differ from all other stroke patients in that *all*, not just part, of the brain may lose its blood supply. This can happen in cases of severe heart failure, certain abnormal heart rhythms, and in some heart attacks when the heart fails to adequately pump blood. Some survivors of *cardiopulmonary resuscitation (CPR)* may also fall into this group.

It was a shock to learn my husband needed surgery to clear blocked arteries in his neck. He felt fine and worked up to the time of his stroke. I guess if you're feeling fine you don't think about going for a physical, but he should have.

Virginia
Age 65

Blood Clotting Abnormalities

Blood clotting abnormalities are responsible for a far less common type of stroke. In these cases, the body's balance between making blood clots and breaking them down shifts, with an increased tendency to make clots that are large enough to cause strokes. Medical scientists are still studying the reasons for this imbalance.

Transient Ischemic Attacks

A *transient ischemic attack* (*TIA*), often called a mini-stroke, is a temporary blockage of an artery. Neurological symptoms go away within twenty-four hours, depending on which artery is blocked. TIAs leave no permanent brain tissue damage. When a person with TIA symptoms arrives in a hospital emergency depart- ment, it may initially be difficult for doctors to tell if the patient is having a TIA or a full-blown stroke. Only time will tell.

I had a brain aneurysm and thought my days were numbered. Only when I got out of intensive care did I think I would live. Recovery is slow, but my energy is coming back each day. I look forward to returning to my part-time job.

Leigh
Age 72

However, TIAs are often "red flag" warnings of strokes to come. An estimated 40 percent of people who suffer TIAs ultimately have strokes, often within a year. People who have several TIAs within a short period of time have a higher risk of developing full-blown strokes. Still, not all TIAs result in stroke. Some people have TIAs that will disappear. Others have TIAs that persist but never progress to stroke. Clearly, medical evaluation at the earliest stage, when brain damage is reversible, is the best way to prevent permanent brain damage.

Brain Lobes: *External View*

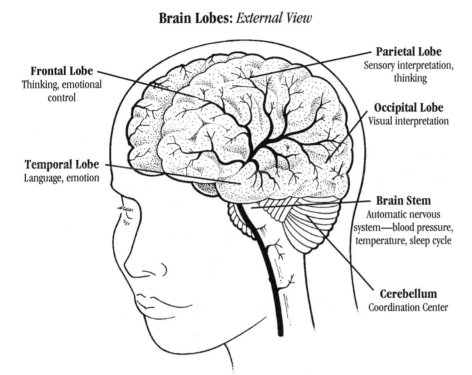

Frontal Lobe
Thinking, emotional
control

Temporal Lobe
Language, emotion

Parietal Lobe
Sensory interpretation,
thinking

Occipital Lobe
Visual interpretation

Brain Stem
Automatic nervous
system—blood pressure,
temperature, sleep cycle

Cerebellum
Coordination Center

Brain Anatomy: The Basics

The upper brain, or *cerebrum,* is divided into two *hemispheres.* The cerebrum contains the *cortical area,* used for thinking, and the *subcortical area,* a complex network of relay centers and linking pathways. Each hemisphere has four separate lobes: frontal, parietal, temporal, and occipital. *Frontal lobes*—located in the front of the brain—control thinking, behavioral functions, and body movement. *Parietal lobes* assist in sensation, concrete thinking (like math), abstract thinking, vision-space orientation, and

Cross Section of Brain

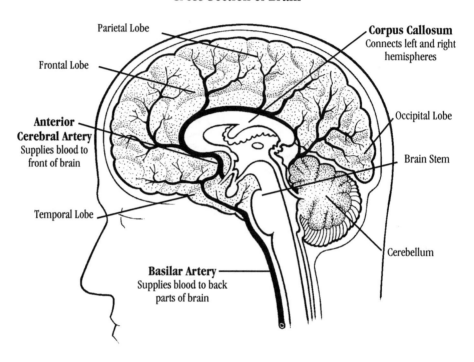

Parietal Lobe

Corpus Callosum
Connects left and right
hemispheres

Frontal Lobe

Occipital Lobe

**Anterior
Cerebral Artery**
Supplies blood to
front of brain

Brain Stem

Temporal Lobe

Cerebellum

Basilar Artery
Supplies blood to back
parts of brain

language. The *temporal lobe* is part of the emotional and memory center and also contains language functions. The *occipital lobe* is the part of the brain that interprets what we see. The back part of the brain, the *cerebellum*, controls balance and coordination. Underneath the cerebrum lies the *brain stem*. It controls involuntary and automatic survival processes we don't need to think about, such as heart rate, body temperature, breathing, sleeping cycles, and the regulation of some hormones.

How Blood Flows to the Brain

Blood moves from the heart to the brain through the large *carotid arteries,* which travel up each side of the neck along the windpipe. Once inside the skull, the carotid arteries divide into front and side branches. These blood vessels supply the front two-thirds of the brain's outer surface. The *vertebrobasilar arteries* travel up and serve this region, as well as the coordination centers and the brain stem.

How the Brain Sends Signals

The wiring of nerves in the brain is complex. Although the two hemispheres of the brain look identical, they handle separate functions. Each hemisphere controls movement and sensation on the *opposite* side of the body. For example, if you accidentally put your left hand under hot running water, the right cerebral cortex interprets the stimulus as pain. To reach for an ice cream cone with your right hand, the left side of the brain generates a signal. The left part of the brain is dominant in right-handed people, while the right portion of the brain is dominant in left-handed individuals.

I was scared that I might not get function back. That haunted me the most. We take small things—like brushing your teeth—for granted, until we can't do them. You don't know for sure what your stroke outcome will be, so you must keep working hard to get better.

Dexter
Age 47

This crossed pattern is not consistent for all brain functions, however. For example, stroke damage to the cerebellum, at the base of the brain, will result in coordination problems on the same side of the body as the brain injury.

Types of Strokes

Strokes are labeled according to the area of the brain that is damaged. For example, if the right hemisphere of the brain loses its blood supply, a right hemisphere stroke occurs. A stroke on the left side of the brain is referred to as a left hemisphere stroke. If an individual suffers a right hemisphere stroke, the left side of the body will be affected. If a stroke occurs in the left cerebrum, the right side of the body will be affected.

Four areas of the brain (artery blood-flow centers) are most commonly affected by stroke. These are listed below, with the deficits that frequently result from them. *Deficits* are deficiencies in mental or physical functions that result from damage to the brain. Common deficits include weakness or paralysis, loss of sensation, problems walking, speaking, and difficulties with *activities of daily living (ADLs)* like dressing, eating, speaking, and grooming.

> *The beginning was the hardest part. I was afraid that I would not get my strength back and that I would be isolated. You have to fight the effects of stroke...go on with your life and keep the faith.*
>
> *Mary*
> *Age 76*

Middle Cerebral Artery Stroke

A stroke occurring in the *middle cerebral artery* may cause:

- loss of feeling on the opposite side of the body
- the arm to usually be weaker than the leg
- significant drooping of the lower half of the face, and drooling
- loss of strength, varying from slight weakness to complete paralysis
- loss of vision, or blind spots

Interior of Brain
View from under chin

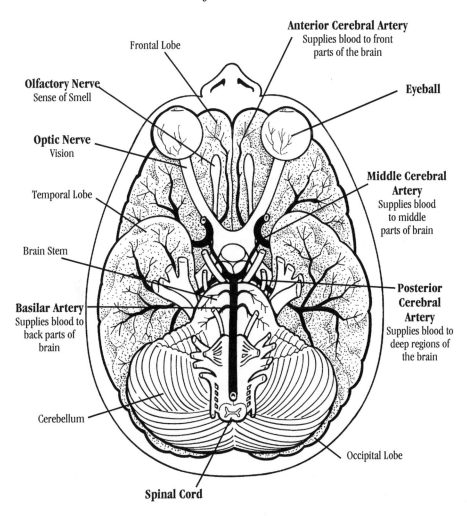

Anterior Cerebral Artery
Supplies blood to front
parts of the brain

Frontal Lobe

Olfactory Nerve
Sense of Smell

Eyeball

Optic Nerve
Vision

Temporal Lobe

**Middle Cerebral
Artery**
Supplies blood
to middle
parts of brain

Brain Stem

Basilar Artery
Supplies blood to
back parts of
brain

**Posterior
Cerebral
Artery**
Supplies blood to
deep regions of
the brain

Cerebellum

Occipital Lobe

Spinal Cord

13

- communication problems, including the inability to understand and produce language
- confusion differentiating between left and right

Anterior Cerebral Artery Stroke

Damage to the *anterior cerebral artery* may cause:
- weakness or paralysis on the opposite side of the body
- the leg to usually be weaker than the arm
- trouble with bowel and bladder control
- opposite-side sensation loss
- intellectual disturbances, including repetitive thought and speech
- disorientation (who and where the patient is and problems understanding aspects of time)
- confusion, forgetfulness, distractibility, and slowed thinking
- an inability to perform tasks when asked, even though the patient has the physical ability to perform the task automatically at other times *(apraxia)*
- facial weakness
- problems with grasp reflex, so strong that the patient cannot let go of objects

Posterior Cerebral Artery Stroke

Strokes occurring in the *posterior cerebral artery* affect the back part of the brain and some of the deep subcortical areas. This artery serves a wide area of brain tissue. Deficit patterns vary depending on which areas are impacted, but may include:
- blind spots on the side opposite where the brain damage occurred

- memory problems and difficulty reading
- severe loss of touch sensation
- burning sensation in the limbs (*thalamic pain syndrome*)
- weakness and involuntary movement disorders
- lack of coordination (*ataxia*)
- cortical blindness, of which the patient is not fully aware

Brain-Stem Stroke

Blockages in the *vertebral and basilar arteries* may damage the brain stem. This particularly vulnerable area includes tightly packed nerve cells, similar to the filaments in a telephone cable. The brain stem controls automatically regulated functions such as heartbeat and breathing. Damage to this area may result in coma or death. Depending on which small blood vessel is blocked, numerous combinations of deficits and syndromes may occur, including:

- sensory loss
- weakness on one side of the body and poor coordination
- swallowing difficulties
- loss of emotional control
- slurred speech
- visual problems, double vision
- dizziness/vertigo
- seizures
- headaches

If the lower portion of the brain stem (*pons*) is deprived of blood, extreme injury can result. Such an injury can create a "locked-in syndrome," in which a patient is virtually "locked" inside the body. The patient is awake but unable to move any limbs. Thinking may be normal, but communication is limited to movement of the eyes and eyelids. The patient becomes a prisoner of his body. Fortunately, this is a rare condition.

Part II

Impairments and Complications Caused by Strokes

2

Cognitive and Sensory Impairments

What is *cognition?* Cognition is an all-encompassing term that refers to the process of thinking and knowing things. It includes awareness, reasoning, remembering, perception, and problem solving. The unique human ability to process information occurs in the outer layer of the brain called the *cerebral cortex.* No one has yet solved all the mysteries of the brain and its amazing capabilities. However, it is a vastly complex organ. Damage to brain tissues can result in a number of changes in cognitive abilities. To further define cognition, we may examine its four basic elements: *perception, intellect, behavior, and emotions.*

Perception

Perception includes depth perception, spatial orientation, and balance. It also includes vision, hearing, taste, smell, and touch. Of all the senses, vision and touch are most often affected by stroke.

Strokes can affect eyesight in several ways. Blind spots may occur when blood clots travel to the back part of the eye and damage the retina. A patient with a blind spot from a right hemisphere stroke may never see a cup of coffee placed on the left side of a breakfast tray. If a blind spot lasts longer than one month after a stroke, it will likely remain a problem. Therapists and nurses teach patients to remember to turn their heads to scan the total environment using their residual vision. Many patients need continued reminders to use this compensatory technique.

After my wife's stroke, her personality changed. She was very angry, and unpleasant to be around. Fortunately, she recovered nicely. My advice to others—try to be understanding and patient.
Gene
Age 67

Damage to other visual pathways in the brain can result in *visual field cuts*. This impairment can be likened to covering half the lenses of your eye glasses with black paint. A patient with a visual field cut may trip over unseen obstacles. Patients with visual field cuts often have a *gaze preference*. They seem to only look in the direction of the vision that remains.

Double vision, or *diplopia*, may result when a stroke affects the brain stem. Some cranial nerves coming out of the brain stem control muscles that move the eyes. If one or more of these nerves is injured, the eyes are not able to move together. This produces two somewhat overlapping images that the brain interprets as double vision. To make only one image reach the brain, some patients will close one eye while others will use an eye patch, alternated daily between the eyes.

Injury to both occipital lobes causes *cortical blindness*, a loss of the ability to interpret visual input. Some individuals may suffer total blindness, while others may be able to distinguish between light and dark. The most peculiar form of cortical blindness is *Anton's Syndrome*, in which a patient is not aware that he is blind. The patient may even insist that all he needs is a pair of glasses to correct his vision.

Touch is the second sense most commonly affected by stroke. Consider the complexity of the sense of touch. If you prick your finger on a pin, a nerve receptor sends a message to the *thalamus*, the brain's "relay" center. From there, the message is sent to the parietal lobe of the brain, and you receive the message that you've stuck your finger. Your reaction is to jerk your finger away from the source of the pain. The entire sequence occurs in an instant. However, a patient who has suffered injury to the parts of the brain responsible for touch sensation may be unaware that his finger was pricked.

When my wife was depressed, I told her I would rather push her around in a wheelchair any day, rather than not have her here with me. I discovered patience I didn't know I had.

Mickey
Age 60

Loss of touch sensation is commonly marked by numbness in the limbs. This makes various tasks more difficult. For example, a patient with a numb hand may crush a paper cup when he picks it up because he can't feel the pressure he's applying. Inability to grasp also interferes with dressing, eating, brushing the hair or teeth, and walking with canes or walkers.

Joint position *(proprioception)* refers to knowing the position of your hand, arm, or leg in space or in relation to other objects. If this sense of joint position is lost, patients can't feel the position of limbs. This creates problems when walking, because patients can't tell when their feet hit the ground. Balance is affected because the ability to feel shifting weight is lost. These patients must learn to use their eyes to judge the relationship between their feet and the floor.

Strokes can cause the loss of touch sensation, temperature—hot and cold, pressure, and vibration.

Intellect

My husband could only remember the distant past. With time, he made improvements. To help him, we would ask him the date, our address, and phone number every day. If he gave the wrong answer, we would tell him and have him repeat it.
Hildegard
Age 48

Intellect, or intelligence, refers to our ability to learn, understand, and act in a purposeful manner. The development of these abilities is influenced by heredity, learning experiences, and motivation. Intellect also includes memory, insight, judgment, orientation, attention span, concentration, problem solving, reasoning/logical thought, abstractions, and ambition. After a stroke, learning may be slower and incomplete because patients are less able to understand. The effects of stroke on the ability to think depend on the area of the brain affected.

Behavior

Behavior is a complex process of actions and responses influenced by our thinking, emotions, and past experiences. Behavior also includes initiative, self-image, decision making, sexuality, and goal-directed behavior. Like other elements of cognition, it's a complex process that can be affected in any number of ways when damage to the brain occurs. For example, a person with brain damage may lose the ability to behave in ways we consider "normal." The result might be a show of anger, agitation, inappropriate laughter or crying, altered sex drive, or sleeping and eating disorders. For example, when serious damage occurs to the frontal lobes of the brain, a patient may show a lack of motivation or may sit for hours unless prompted to act.

Emotions

Damage to the parts of the brain that control *emotions* can result in personality changes. If the ability to control emotions is lost, patients may display emotionally extreme behaviors. They may cry over situations that would make other people happy. Other times, they may laugh inappropriately—at a funeral, for example. Such poor emotional control is known as *emotional lability*. It can be confusing to the patient and to observers since the patient's feelings will not be matched by his behaviors. To clarify the real emotion experienced by the patient, caregivers should simply ask the patient to describe what he is feeling, and compare this with the demonstrated behavior. Families might try changing the topic or distracting the patient to breakup this emotion.

I depended on using humor against becoming depressed. Regaining my balance and learning to walk was physically and mentally very tough.

Owen
Age 66

Anger often accompanies personality changes. Patients who previously had loving and gentle manners may now seem very angry. This may be due in part to the overwhelming frustration of handling all the changes caused by the stroke. On the other hand, injury for some patients may have the opposite effect. They instead may become agreeable and cheerful. Often, these personality changes seem impulsive or even bizarre.

Of all the emotional changes that stroke patients may experience, *depression* is one that certainly deserves special mention. Understandably, the effects of a stroke can spark major depression. Imagine that you have spent weeks or months in a hospital, unable to function as you normally would. As the mental fog lifts, you realize that no matter how hard you try to imitate a therapist's movements, your arm and leg just won't move. The chance of ever walking around the house seems an improbability. Negotiating steps into your home is unthinkable. You choke when you try to eat because your swallowing mechanism isn't working. Everything you do from the time you wake until you go to sleep requires someone else's help. No one seems to understand anything you say. Likewise, the words spoken to you seem like gibberish. Your mind becomes preoccupied with and then consumed by thoughts of never going home...never living with your spouse...never again experiencing physical love. You cry uncontrollably as you reflect on your losses. This is an accurate picture of how depression can set in after a stroke.

It was frustrating getting the diagnosis made. At times, we had problems communicating with the medical and nursing staff. Part of the problem is just not knowing the right questions to ask.

Paula
Age 43

In the early stages of injury to the brain, some people aren't really aware that they are unable to perform basic daily tasks. Their moods may be pleasant. Others may deny problems and deficits during much of their rehabilitation as inpatients. This may be a natural defense against the stress of such a major health problem. However, later on, depression may ensue as patients begin to grieve the loss of functions like speech and walking.

Depression focuses energy and attention on the problem rather than recovery. Patients may "shut down" and not participate in therapies. If the depression is severe enough, their physical performance may continue to decline over time.

Some studies conservatively estimate that about 8 percent of new stroke patients suffer minor depression, while up to 15 percent experience major depression. Other studies indicate an overall 40 percent rate of depression. Although research is not definitive, it seems that damage to the left side of the brain more frequently results in depression than damage to the right side.

Depression is a deep sadness, a feeling of hopelessness and helplessness. It can manifest itself in any of the following symptoms:

- low energy
- loss of interest in people or things that were once enjoyable
- crying for no apparent reason
- agitation for no apparent reason
- decrease in body movements as the patient withdraws from the world
- sense of guilt or desire to die (perhaps due to feeling like a burden to others)
- sleep disturbances (insomnia or excessive sleeping)
- changes in eating patterns (eating too much or not enough)
- weight changes
- vague complaints of body pains without other medical explanation

Even medical professionals sometimes have difficulty identifying depression because the symptoms may be masked by a patient's dulled levels of consciousness, fatigue from therapy, altered sleeping and eating abilities, and the inability to communicate. People close to a patient who acts depressed should contact a physician immediately, especially if the patient expresses suicidal thoughts.

There are several ways to treat depression. Psychiatrists, psychologists, or counselors may discuss depression with patients and provide counseling to help them adjust to the new disability. This type of help may not be appropriate for all people. A patient who is barely alert or who has a communication impairment, for example, will unlikely benefit from counseling.

Antidepressant medications, prescribed for varying periods of time, are usually started at low doses and increased (if necessary) based on a patient's response. Medical supervision ensures effectiveness and monitors possible side effects.

Families and friends can also play a major role in a patient's recovery from depression and in rehabilitation. It is a fact that strong family support increases a patient's chances for improvement. Family members may participate in support groups and in various therapies. Patients often respond more favorably to family than to therapists, and such team effort is necessary for patients to realize gains. Families can encourage patients to perform activities, giving them a feeling of success and self-esteem, which usually motivates them to progress to more difficult tasks. Patients who formerly rose to life's challenges should be reminded by loved ones that they can use the same determination to battle the effects of stroke.

3

Speech and Language Disruptions

Most of us take speaking for granted. It seems simple, for we learned how to speak in early childhood. But in truth, speech is a remarkably complex process. Speech starts with a thought in the brain. Then the brain sends signals to nerves that move the mouth, tongue, throat, voice box, and lungs. The result is what we call speech or language. We can also control our tone of voice, volume, and the speed of our speech. Physical gestures add yet another dimension to our communication skills. A stroke may damage brain tissues that control complex communication functions.

For stroke patients who have suffered a lot of brain damage, virtually all means of communication may fail. Other patients may not lose much capability, but they may be so drowsy from medications that they aren't able to pay attention long enough to understand communication. Or, the effects of the stroke may dampen their level of consciousness enough to prevent communication. For patients at the other end of the spectrum, a good deal of recovery may be possible. Recovery of speech, however, may be as unpredictable as other types of functional recovery. The best way to assess improvement is to analyze trends over a period of time and to then determine if further therapy can be beneficial.

Aphasia

When a stroke causes damage to the left hemisphere of the brain, a patient almost always has *aphasia*, difficulty and hesitancy forming words and difficulty understanding language. Aphasia can affect any aspect of our ability to communicate—speech, comprehension, and gestures. The effects of aphasia can vary from patient to patient. Some patients may be completely unable to speak or may have limited vocabularies that may not mean anything to the rest of us. Other aphasic patients may be able to speak but do not understand what they are saying or what others are saying to them. It is as if they were suddenly dropped into another country, where a foreign language was being spoken. Still other patients may understand speech but be unable to think of the words to respond.

My speech problems tend to get worse with stress and fatigue. At first, I couldn't read, write, or speak. I was lucky to recover quickly. I was back at work in two months, but needed help from friends.

Karen
Age 39

Patients with aphasia are initially confused by their inability to understand and form words. This can lead to panic and anxiety, and for some, depression. Psychiatrists and psychologists may evaluate these patients, but counseling success may be limited by the language barrier. On the other hand, some patients may not experience these negative emotions because they may lack insight into the fact that others do not understand what they say. These people may remain content even though their language deficits are severe.

Problems common to most types of aphasia include an inability to process long words and infrequently used words. Family and friends should use short, commonly used words when speaking with, or writing to, an aphasic stroke patient. It helps to give messages slowly and clearly with gestures and repetition. Family and caregivers can also learn to recognize that patients with speech difficulties may use subtle variations in tone to communicate more effectively. It is helpful to keep tissues close at hand to help patients who drool when they speak due to their loss of facial muscle strength.

Patients may be distracted by surrounding movement and noise, so it is useful to eliminate the source (TV, radio, a crowded room) when communicating with them. An alphabet board or pencil and paper may be used to spell out words.

I'm lucky to have survived a cerebellar stroke. The most frustrating thing was regaining my speech. I knew what I wanted to say, but the words would not come. After months of therapy, I made a good recovery.
Ramona
Age 67

Types of Aphasia

Global Aphasia

The most damaging language disturbance is called *global aphasia*. Patients with global aphasia seem to understand very few words, either spoken or written. They may be completely unable to speak, or their speech may be hesitant and broken. Most are unable to repeat words. If they can speak, they may have a limited vocabulary and may not make sense to the rest of us. Sometimes, profanities are the only words a patient with global aphasia can utter. This may happen to previously even-tempered individuals, who for some unknown reason are capable of producing only these words. This can be disheartening to family and friends. But, even though it is not socially desirable, it a good sign the patient is able to form some words.

Global aphasia can limit chances for successful rehabilitation since both the ability to produce language and understand it are seriously impaired. If global aphasia does not improve, patients may require considerable help from family or other caregivers. In addition to having difficulty in relearning ADLs, patients tend to have more problems with bladder control, in part because they can't communicate their needs. With time and repetition, the hope is that these patients will eventually be able to perform all or part of ADLs automatically. Some patients may relearn self-care skills but may not really comprehend why they are doing them.

My husband has shown a positive attitude and sense of humor since having his stroke. His functions are slowly improving. Some times he can't recall a specific word and substitutes another one that sounds similar. He keeps working at it.
Marilyn
Age 59

Broca's Aphasia

Patients with *Broca's aphasia* know what they want to say and try to say it but are unable to find the right words. The impairment may be mild or severe. These patients may have some problems with comprehension, although usually not severe problems. Communication can best be facilitated by asking a patient questions that can be answered with "yes" or "no." Speech therapists may use a technique known as *melodic intonation therapy,* in which familiar songs are used to tap into parts of the brain that can overcome this speech deficit. Pictorial communication boards can help some patients.

Wernicke's Aphasia

Individuals with *Wernicke's aphasia* can neither make sense of what is being said to them nor monitor what they are saying. Damage to speech centers in the back part of the brain causes this deficit. Speech may be very fluent but may not make much sense at times, even though grammar may be correct and the speech not slurred. The ability to repeat words and name objects is often impaired. Some patients may make up nonsense words that have meanings only to them. Treatment involves trying to increase a patient's understanding of what he hears and improving speech output. Varying levels of improvement are usually seen with both Wernicke's and Broca's aphasia.

Even though my husband has aphasia, I include him in conversations and have others speak to him, not around him. He works crossword puzzles to keep his intellect sharp. Don't isolate the stroke survivor. Reinforce self-worth and include them in decision-making.

Rosemary
Age 70

Dysarthria

Dysarthria is slurred speech. It results from damage to the nerves that serve the voice box, tongue, and mouth. Usually patients are able to say words and understand language but their articulation (mouth and tongue movement) is poor. Patients also may not be able to control their breathing well enough to produce loud vocal sounds, and slurring may result. They should be encouraged to take a deep breath before trying to speak. Brain damage may cause their speech to sound hypernasal or monotone.

Speech pathologists teach patients overarticulation exercises, which involve overexaggerating tongue and mouth movements while speaking. A mirror may be used to help visualize facial muscles as words are formed. Patients who tend to speak too quickly need to be reminded to speak slowly to prevent further slurring of words.

Speech Therapy Evaluation

Speech pathologists may need to spend a fair amount of time with aphasic patients before the extent of damage to their communication abilities can be determined. An evaluation typically involves assessing:

- the ability to speak
- hearing
- auditory comprehension (the ability to understand what is said)
- the ability to follow both simple and complex spoken and gestural commands
- thinking abilities (memory, abstraction, organization skills, decision-making skills)
- the ability to move the cheeks, tongue, and lips (to check for weakness or paralysis)
- writing skills
- reading comprehension

Based on this analysis, speech pathologists will attempt to design strategies to help patients overcome speech deficits. To observing family and friends, there may be times in the course of speech therapy that the activities—like matching colors and patterns or words to pictures—may seem silly or simplistic. But for stroke patients, these tasks may be as difficult to learn as they were in childhood. This truly is a process of starting over. Communication foundations need to be established before more complex tasks may be learned. It is important for friends and family to be supportive of patients during this time, rather than judgmental or critical. Any lack of progress while learning skills is probably due to brain damage rather than laziness or lack of effort.

In addition to therapy, some patients may improve as a result of the brain's *plasticity,* the ability of undamaged brain tissue to take over functions previously handled by a part that was damaged. In some left cortical strokes where language ability is disrupted, the right cortical brain may assume some language functions. Research indicates that the left frontal lobe may also increase its activity to help recover language. A chemical called *synaptophysin* actually increases in both sides of the brain after a stroke and may assist in recovery by strengthening the connections among nerve cells. Left-handed people may have a better chance to recover from aphasia. Why? It seems there is a spreading out of language functions within the brain, and some parts of the brain may sustain less damage.

> *Early on, my mother could hear what we said, but could not speak. It was like playing charades. When she first started talking, she could say just one or two words. The rest was gibberish. We learned to laugh. I think the sense of humor helped.*
>
> *Larry*
> *Age 50*

Accessory Communication

In addition to speech therapy, some patients may need help with accessory communication skills. For example, some patients may need eyeglasses to help with vision problems. Special glasses are available for those who may have double vision, or diplopia. Others may need hearing aids to improve hearing. Some patients may need dentures. Teeth are important to the pronunciation of words, and a good set of fitted dentures can go a long way toward correcting slurring. If the ability to write or gesture is impaired as the result of weakened arm muscles, an occupational therapist may help patients learn to write as well as gesture with their nondominant hands.

4

Hemiplegia

The most common impairment resulting from a stroke is *hemiplegia*, a weakness on one side of the body. It can affect the entire side, or only an arm or a leg. The weakness will affect the side opposite the brain damage. If the stroke injured the right side of the brain, the weakness or paralysis will be on the left side of the body, and vice versa.

Patients may show a variety of weakness patterns immediately after a stroke. For some, a limb may be weak, even totally limp. Others may experience a progression of weakness. Initially, the fingers and hand may become weak, then the paralysis may move up the entire arm. Interestingly, recovery of function often seems to occur in the reverse order, with the fingers being the last to recover movement.

Apraxia and Neglect

Some patients have *apraxia*, the inability to move a limb when asked. Basically, the brain is not able to plan out the requested movement. Repetitive training may produce some progress in cases of apraxia.

Others may have a problem with *neglect,* lack of awareness or recognition of some parts of the environment. A patient with neglect may not only ignore the side of the body that is weak but also that side of his world. For example, if the weakness appears on his left side, he may not eat food from the left side of his plate. This condition creates problems for people who are relearning how to feed, dress, or groom themselves. Women may put makeup on only one side of the face, while men may show up half-shaved. In mild cases, patients may understand their lack of awareness and can compensate. However, in a severe case, a patient may be unable to tell the difference between his own arm and someone else's. Neglect may also affect mobility. Patients may walk or steer their wheelchairs into objects they don't see on their "neglected" sides.

The toughest part was learning to walk again. It was difficult because my feet felt stiff. I never doubted I would make improvements. After several strokes, I understand the key is to keep working hard and don't give up.
Elzra
Age 60

Recovering Muscle Strength

Strength recovery is the process of re-establishing connections from the brain to the muscles. The recovery from muscle weakness can range from almost unnoticeable to regaining normal strength. As signals from the brain begin to reach the muscles, a recovering patient develops voluntary motion. Muscles may gain strength with time, healing, and exercise, but most stroke patients will suffer some level of permanent weakness.

The goal of therapy is to restore as much strength and movement as possible. But, before therapy exercises can be prescribed for weak limbs, therapists must first evaluate the patient's muscle strength, joint range of motion, balance, coordination, vision, hearing, and ability to understand instructions. Once accomplished, exercises can begin for each major muscle group. The intensity of exercise increases as muscles develop, improving both strength and coordination.

Therapists test muscle strength and grade it on a 0 to 5 scale, as shown in Table 1. Then, exercise is prescribed based on strength and ability to move. For example, an arm with a grade of 2/5 may move if placed in a position where the effect of gravity is eliminated. The same arm may not be able to lift against gravity, so the use of resistance weights would not only be futile but dangerous. A muscle must have some strength before active-motion exercises can help.

Table 1. Muscle Strength Grades

Grade 0/5	No muscle motion.
Grade 1/5 (trace)	A muscle moves.
Grade 2/5 (poor)	A muscle moves a joint if gravity is eliminated.
Grade 3/5 (fair)	A muscle moves a joint against gravity.
Grade 4/5 (good)	A muscle moves a joint against resistance.
Grade 5/5 (normal)	A muscle moves with normal strength.

If a person develops too much *spasticity,* tightening of muscles and joints as the result of abnormal signals from the brain, an arm or leg brace may be a partial solution. Use of a tilt table can also help stretch the feet and heel cords using the patient's own body weight as resistance. These exercises are usually done along with range of motion exercises. Powerful muscle tone can interfere with voluntary movement. *Tone* refers to the resistance of a muscle when someone else moves the joint near the muscle. Patients may develop excessive tone as a result of spasticity. In the arm, spasticity usually brings the arm joints into a bent (flexed) position. Spasticity in the leg usually extends the limb joints. Arms may also be extended and legs may also be bent. Regardless, spasticity makes it harder to perform desired motions. This slows progress toward achieving ADLs.

Walking required much patience and determination. New accomplishments do not come daily. Patients like to hear praise even for small accomplishments. On days a patient seems uncooperative, do not pressure him. Try to be sensitive to his feelings.

Mary Jo
Age 73

Patients with tendencies to lean to one side and those who have poor balance may find a full-length mirror placed at the end of parallel bars a helpful source of visual feedback. Some of these patients have *pusher syndrome.* They overbalance by pushing with the muscles on the stronger side, tilting them toward the weak side. This is a safety concern if the action is strong and persistent, because it can cause falling episodes.

Joint function is also important to muscle strength. Joints must be flexible for us to move our limbs. Therapists may say that a joint has *functional range*, which means there is enough joint mobility to perform everyday tasks. Range of motion and stretching exercises can prevent *joint contractures*, where soft tissue shortens and prevents a full range of movement of the limbs.

A therapist may also use passive range of motion exercises, moving parts of the body for a patient who is unable to perform the motion independently. Also, fluid buildup in the hands, caused by immobility, may make it difficult for a patient to grasp objects. Occupational therapists may massage the fingers and hands to keep swelling at a minimum. Compression gloves also serve this purpose and prevent more swelling.

Regaining Coordination

Lack of coordination is especially noticeable in strokes affecting the cerebellum and its pathways. The cerebellum, located at the back of the brain, is the coordination center. To make a coordinated movement, the brain tells which muscles to move. For example, to scratch the nose, the brain instructs one set of muscles to contract while the opposite set relaxes. After a stroke, what once seemed a thoughtless process has suddenly become a major project. If the brain can't coordinate its signals, the stroke patient may poke his eye instead of scratching the nose. *Inhibition* is a brain signal that tells a muscle not to move. Damaged inhibition causes more muscles than necessary to move.

Even though my father suffered paralysis on his left side, he never gave up hope of getting back to the golf course, even if he had to play with one hand. When he finally took a few steps with a walker, we were elated, and reminded him of how far he had come.

Karen
Age 38

To regain coordination, persistence and the repetition of exercises cannot be overemphasized. Why? It is believed that to produce muscle coordination, a movement must be repeated hundreds of thousands of times. Experts believe that motor loops develop in the brain as an activity is repeated and learned. These motor loops are called *engrams.* A normal brain performs hundreds of thousands of correctly performed signals to achieve coordination. Many types of strokes injure engram pathways, and they must be rebuilt through repetition. This means practice is important. Caregivers can help patients with exercises outside therapy sessions, increasing their potential for progress.

How Long Will It Take?

I'm very frustrated by the weakness in my left side, but I hope to get back enough strength to walk. I am grateful to have such a supportive family. They are willing to do whatever it takes to help me recover.

Robert
Age 46

The amount of time it takes to regain muscle strength is unpredictable. If a comparison were made of all stroke patients with damage to the same area of the brain, the amount of time needed for recovery would vary greatly. For muscles to work, signals from the brain must reach them again. Often, the signals may reconnect once swelling decreases and/or when undamaged portions of the brain take over the functions of damaged cells. Brain scans help determine the amount of damaged tissue, which in turn helps the medical team guess how much recovery to expect. But even scientific tools and doctors' best estimates can be wrong.

Rehabilitation professionals tend to agree that patients who have the potential to make functional gains do better if therapy is started soon after a stroke. There are different schools of thought on how much recovery is possible. One study of stroke patients in Copenhagen showed that, by the end of three months (including rehabilitation), 95 percent of patients recovered the most functional recovery they could ever hope for. On the other hand, the medical community is recognizing new studies that cite cases in which improvement is shown at six months and beyond. Authors of one study report cases of improvement seven years after a stroke. Accordingly, there is a place for rehabilitation therapy beyond just the first few weeks after a stroke.

Even after rehabilitation has ended, and all the physical recovery has taken place, there still may be the chance to learn how to cope with the disability.

5

Dysphagia

When brain damage affects control of the muscles in the throat, cheek, jaw, and tongue, *dysphagia*—difficulty with swallowing—may result. About half the people who have strokes have some problems with swallowing. For these individuals, eating may be troublesome. With dysphagia, any of the swallowing stages can be affected.

Stages of Swallowing

In a normal swallow, once a bite of food (*bolus*) nears the voice box, a flap of tissue (*epiglottis*) comes down to cover the windpipe (*trachea*) to let the bolus slide past into the body's swallowing passage (*esophagus*). There is a danger zone where the breathing and swallowing tubes meet. Even for people with normal swallowing abilities, food and fluids will sometimes slip into the trachea rather than the esophagus. *Penetration* is the term used to describe what happens when food lodges near or slightly below the vocal cords. If the bolus, such as a piece of poorly chewed meat, is big enough, it may stick in the airway and block it. At best, this is a scary situation. At worst, a patient may choke and die unless the obstruction is quickly removed. Loss of control of the bolus may cause food to pocket in the cheeks and spill backward into the open airway.

The Stages of Swallowing Food

Oral stage	Food/fluid is taken into the mouth. Chewing makes food/fluid into a ball (*bolus*) to present to the back of the throat.
Pharyngeal stage	Food/fluid is pushed down past the protected voice box.
Esophageal stage	Food/fluid is moved by muscular waves down the esophagus and past a bend into the stomach.

Aspiration

Among the most serious complications resulting from dysphagia is *aspiration,* the suction of food or fluid into the lungs. Aspiration occurs when a bolus washes mouth and throat bacteria past the vocal cords and into the lungs. This can result in *aspiration pneumonia,* which can be mild or severe. One of the frightening aspects of dysphagia is *silent aspiration.* A patient may appear normal while eating and drinking but has sucked food into the lungs. Up to 40 percent of stroke patients are believed to experience silent aspiration. This seems to be a particular problem in patients who have damage to the brain stem. A complicated set of motions, involving several nerves that originate in the brain stem, are involved in transporting food.

Silent aspiration can also occur when the protective cough mechanism disappears. A sensitive patch of tissue exists at the bottom of the windpipe where it branches off to each lung. If food or fluid touches this area, the normal reaction will produce a strong cough reflex to force out the foreign substance. If this reflex is not working, patients may show no signs of choking or coughing even while pneumonia-causing materials are entering the lungs.

Right after my mom's stroke, I saw her take a sip of fluid. It all ran right back out of her mouth. It was really frightening. I wondered if she would ever be able to eat again. We're grateful that she did recover.

Rod
Age 47

Other problems can also cause aspiration. In the esophageal stage of swallowing, the inability of muscles to propel a bolus into the stomach may cause food to come back up the esophagus and be sucked into the trachea. Medication may be needed to push the bolus down into the stomach. An operation may be needed to open up the top of the swallowing tube to allow food to pass into it if the ring of muscle at the top of the swallowing tube is so tight it can't open at the right time. Some patients may require surgical placement of a tube in the windpipe, called a *tracheostomy tube*. This tube protects the airway and gives immediate access if the lungs need to be suctioned. Sometimes, aspiration may occur even if a tracheostomy tube is in place. If a patient has a delayed swallowing reflex, a bolus may lodge in the back of the throat. Bits of it may then fall into the unprotected airway. Sometimes, the ring of muscle at the top of the swallowing tube doesn't open up. The bolus has nowhere to go except around the airway.

Diagnosing Dysphagia

Dysphagia isn't always obvious. Dysphagia caused by a brainstem stroke may be present even when a brain scan looks normal. If silent aspiration is suspected, it is best to do a *videofluoroscopy*, or a *modified barium swallow test*. This X-ray test shows food and fluid movement during a swallow. Rather than producing a single picture, an X-ray video camera tapes a patient swallowing food of different consistencies. The various stages of swallowing may be observed. Based upon test results, doctors and speech therapists decide whether the patient may safely eat different types of foods or drink fluids. The test identifies food consistencies that might cause problems. It is important to understand that this test is not infallible. Test results might vary from day to day. The swallowing reflex might be fine if the patient is having a good day. On another day, perhaps when the patient is tired, swallowing limitations and a greater risk of aspiration may show up. Using the videofluoroscopy results, the medical team will try to make reasonable clinical decisions.

I was devastated when I had a stroke. It really changed my life. I learned to focus on one goal at a time...it helped me make progress. Remember, set a goal and therapy... therapy.

Don
Age 72

Therapies for Dysphagia

A speech therapist may decide that a patient may benefit from swallowing therapy. Therapy goals include the ability to ingest adequate amounts of food and fluids, the ability to prevent aspiration pneumonia and airway obstructions through safe swallowing, and finding a diet the patient can tolerate. Puréed foods and thick liquids often provide the safest initial nutrition because they are substantial enough for the patient to hold in the mouth until it is time to swallow. Food of regular consistency may be tried later when the patient is able to chew and swallow well enough to prevent airway blockages.

Speech pathologists can help patients learn to chew and swallow if these functions are impaired or lost. Exercises include bolus control using the lips and tongue while food is in the mouth. Videofluoroscopy may indicate that a chin-tilt maneuver may help use gravity to keep the bolus at the front of the mouth until the patient can initiate the swallow. Sometimes trying to suck ice cream through a straw strengthens muscles. The patient may be taught to check for leftover food by sweeping the mouth with a finger.

Having a stroke can bring a drastic change in your way of living. Through my therapy and educational support of therapists, doctors, and family members, I am able to get back to my way of living.

Anna

Age 84

Rehabilitation for the pharyngeal stage, when food and fluid are in the throat, often centers around speeding up the swallowing reflex. This reflex should normally take about one second. But in some patients it may be delayed for many seconds, or it may not occur at all. Therapists may try *thermal stimulation.* Here, a long-handled mirror, like those used by dentists, is cooled in ice water and placed at the sides of the inner throat. This is a simple technique for caregivers to learn. Thermal stimulation improves swallowing by increasing the speed of the swallowing reflex.

Occupational therapists may teach patients the mechanics of getting food and fluids from the meal tray to the mouth.

Dysphagia

They may watch for patients who eat impulsively and teach them to eat more slowly and safely. Sometimes special adaptive equipment makes moving food from the dish to the mouth easier. A patient may also learn to use his nondominant hand. Dietitians can help develop the right consistencies of food and fluids and monitor other factors like salt or calorie restrictions.

Like other forms of therapy, treatments to improve swallowing will include some successes and some failures. Again, outcomes are hard to predict. Much of the progress depends upon the patient's ability to cooperate and learn.

Alternative Feeding Methods

Patients who are unable to swallow food of any consistency may be restricted from taking any type of nutrition by mouth. This is called keeping patients *NPO*, meaning "nothing by mouth."

Other patients may have the ability to swallow, but brain damage prevents them from eating enough to receive adequate nutrition. In either case, patients must be fed to prevent malnutrition or dehydration.

Nasogastric Tubes

Until swallowing problems can be fully evaluated, doctors may insert a *nasogastric tube*, or *NG tube*. This flexible plastic tube is inserted through the nose and threaded through the swallowing tube into the stomach. An NG tube can provide a patient with a means to take in water and a special feeding solution. The tube bypasses the lungs, preventing risk of aspiration pneumonia. Insertion of an NG tube is usually done at bedside while the patient is awake. It is an uncomfortable procedure, for the tube stings the back of the nose and throat as it is inserted. But once installed, it is usually not too uncomfortable. The NG tube will need to be replaced if a patient intentionally or unintentionally pulls it out. Even if a videofluoroscopy shows that the patient is able to eat some types of food, an NG tube may still be needed to help supplement nutrition.

Intravenous Feedings

Patients may initially receive nourishment through a tube inserted into a vein in the arm, an *intravenous line.* Intravenous (IV) solutions, and some medications, are contained in bags. The solution is slowly pumped into the veins. IV solutions may irritate the veins and limit the amount of nutrition that may be given. Use of IVs is usually temporary unless there is a problem with the stomach or intestines, in which case a *central IV line* may be needed. The central IV line is placed into one of the large veins at the base of the neck. Since larger veins are used, more concentrated nutritional solutions may be given.

Gastrostomy Tubes

Another feeding alternative is the *gastrostomy tube*, also called a *G-tube* or *PEG tube*. It requires a minor surgical procedure, usually lasting less than thirty minutes, during which a flexible tube is inserted directly through the abdominal wall and into the stomach. The G-tube replaces an older method of surgically implanting a feeding tube, which caused more infection and bleeding and required more sedation. In most cases, the G-tube is usable in a day or two. Until then, the patient is fed intravenous fluids.

A G-tube is a good alternative for many patients. At least one study suggests there are fewer deaths associated with the use of G-tubes than with the continual use of NG tubes. An NG tube may still allow contents of the stomach to track back up the esophagus and into the back of the throat, where aspiration may occur.

Because G-tubes create a surgical opening in the abdominal wall, the cut tissue may become infected. Antibiotics are prescribed if a patient develops a skin infection at the insertion site. In extreme cases, the tube may need to be removed. Rarely, some of the stomach fluids may leak out and irritate the skin. Use of special skin barriers may prevent this.

Depending on the need, the G-tube may be used for either a short period of time or long-term. Often, over the course of several weeks to several months, another videofluoroscopy may be performed to see if the swallowing function has improved. If so, the patient may try orally taking some food and fluid. Many families insist that the G-tube come out as soon as a swallowing test looks normal. This can prove to be a mistake due to the test's limitations. It is usually better to leave the tube in until the patient proves, over time, that he can swallow well without developing pneumonia, coughing, or choking.

Removing the G-tube is a simple procedure. In most cases, the hole shrinks and closes on its own. Rarely, doctors will need to loop a few stitches around the hole to help it close. Expect a small, button-sized scar to remain after the tube comes out. Overall, G-tubes have been of great benefit to patients of all diagnoses who need them.

6

Bladder, Bowel, and Sexual Problems

B owel, bladder, and sexual dysfunctions are some of the most challenging and discouraging issues a stroke patient and caregivers can face. Loss of any of these functions can produce feelings of depression and inadequacy. To the patient, these dysfunctions may represent "badges" of disability. Friends and family need to provide support and encourage loved ones to regain as much normal activity as possible.

Bladder Problems

Loss of bladder control, or *bladder incontinence*, shows up as urination or leakage that is out of one's control. Incontinence tends to occur more often in women because of the effects of childbirth and because the urine tube, or *urethra*, is much shorter in women than in men.

Normally, the bladder stretches like a balloon and stores urine made in the kidneys. Then, when it is filled, signals from the bladder travel to the brain to inform it that there is a need to *void*, or urinate. When we reach the toilet, the brain coordinates relaxation of the bladder neck, allowing the bladder to contract and eliminate the urine.

Stroke damage to these nerve pathways can impact bladder functions in several ways. First, a patient may have lost the sensations that signal a need to urinate. Predictably, the patient becomes incontinent. Second, the bladder may send false signals. A patient may feel like he has to go to the bathroom frequently but in reality does not need to urinate. In yet other cases, a urine buildup may push urine back up into the kidneys and cause damage or infection. This may occur if a muscle tightens at the bladder outlet. Rather than emptying the urine normally, it creates a backup. Third, problems with urinating will occur if the bladder loses its tone. It will act like a passive sack and will retain urine. In this situation, a person may be incontinent only after the bladder fills up with extremely large volumes. Medications are available to help add tone to the bladder. Finally, in the early stages of a stroke, communication impairments may cause bladder problems. A patient may be unable to let caregivers know that he needs to urinate. The patient may not be able to delay urinating long enough for someone to understand and assist him.

Initially, I had poor bladder control and needed medication to help me until my body could heal. I hated therapy at first, but later realized the value of putting in a hard day at it. My husband and I are closer now because of all the support he has given me.

Chris
Age 40

Additional help for bladder problems may be sought from *urologists*, specialists who work with the urinary system. As part of an evaluation, a urologist will study a patient's voiding pattern. The specialist may examine *urodynamics* to test the bladder's ability to expand and contract and its volume. The test also determines whether the patient can feel the bladder filling and the contraction of the bladder neck and sphincter muscles. Using this information, the doctor may prescribe medications.

Urinary Tract Infections

In a normal bladder, few bacteria are present, certainly not enough to make someone sick. Additionally, the bladder has an inner lining of *mucus,* a thick, sticky substance that traps bacteria. However, if the bladder retains urine, more bacteria than usual may collect. Sometimes germs may get past this layer and enter the bloodstream. If this happens, a person may become very sick with a high temperature, loss of appetite, chills, sweating, and even a dangerous drop in blood pressure. This group of symptoms is called *urosepsis* and requires antibiotics, often given intravenously. It is the most severe *urinary tract infection (UTI)* involving either the bladder or the kidneys.

A more common but less serious UTI occurs when germs are confined to the bladder. Symptoms include low-grade fever, burning on urination, frequent urination, and cloudy, foul-smelling urine. Some of these infections may seem to cause incontinence. However, it may be instead that the germs irritate the bladder wall enough, causing the bladder to contract repeatedly as a protective reaction to get rid of the germs. This type of UTI may be handled with oral antibiotics or intravenous antibiotics, depending on how sick a person is and which germ is causing the infection.

Doctors diagnose UTIs by evaluating symptoms. They may also screen a urine sample for signs of infection, such as white blood cells and bacteria. The lab may use a urine specimen to grow the bacteria and test antibiotics to see which ones will work effectively. This may take several days and lead to changes in antibiotic treatment. If symptoms are minimal, doctors may prefer to wait until the urine culture grows identifiable bacteria before they choose an antibiotic.

Managing a Neurogenic Bladder

A *neurogenic bladder* is one that is working poorly due to nerve damage in the brain. The goal of treatment is to allow sufficient emptying and storage of urine. Accordingly, fluid intake may be limited so that the bladder doesn't overfill. Patients still unable to void on their own must have their bladders passively drained by care staff. This involves intermittent use of a *catheter,* a tube inserted up the urethra into the bladder, to drain the urine. This is an *intermittent catheterization program (ICP).* For some patients, an *indwelling catheter* (left in place) may be needed to drain urine into a bag worn under the clothing, attached to a leg, or placed at the side of a bed. Statistically, an indwelling catheter causes more urinary tract infections than the intermittent catheter, but in some circumstances the former may be the only practical solution. Less commonly, a urologist may insert a *suprapubic catheter,* or *SP catheter.* The tube is placed in a surgically made hole low in the abdomen, just above the pubic bone. Either catheter may introduce bacteria into the bladder. With any type of catheter, it is important to maintain good fluid intake to help flush bacteria from the bladder.

Bowel Problems

During the process of digestion and elimination, the food we eat enters the stomach and moves through the small and large intestines. The waste products then pass on to the rectum. When the walls of the rectum stretch and fill with stool material, a signal sent to the brain encourages us to find a bathroom. But, just as some individuals have bladder control problems as a result of stroke, others have problems with bowel incontinence.

To make it through a stroke, both patient and family must have faith that you can handle it. My husband can only walk short distances; the lack of movement makes his bowels sluggish. I think it's important to pray a lot and get away for short periods to take time for yourself.

Norma
Age 61

The goal of bowel management is to keep the bowels moving regularly and to help patients avoid spilling stool contents between evacuations. Bowel-control problems may result from the inability to hold the stool inside the rectum or from the inability to communicate the need to use the toilet.

Constipation

Bowels may become sluggish and *constipation* may result when the body is limited to bed rest. Once a patient gets out of bed and becomes more active, especially when walking, constipation often resolves or lessens. However, if one stays inactive, stool may accumulate and become impacted. This may require much more medication to push the stool through to the rectum. Some impactions may require removal of the stool by a professional using a finger inserted in the rectum. Although not a pleasant experience, this can be quite effective.

Stool softener is a medication that mixes water from the digestive tract with the stool to make it softer. This makes it easier and less irritating to have a bowel movement. Stool softeners may also be useful if a person has *hemorrhoids,* enlarged blood vessels in the rectal area. Hemorrhoids may be painful during some bowel movements, especially if the stool is hard.

There are several types of *laxatives.* *Bulk laxatives* are usually made of powdered fiber, formed into tablets or mixed into water or juice and swallowed. These laxatives absorb water in the digestive tract, which in turn swells the fiber. The volume of the fiber stretches the rectal walls and comes closest to reproducing the body's natural function. *Stimulant laxatives* cause bowel movements by irritating the digestive tract and forcing the gut to push waste toward the rectum. However, if these laxatives are used too often, the bowels may become dependent on them. Stimulant laxatives can be given orally or rectally, as a suppository or enema. Use of mineral oil as a laxative should be avoided in patients with swallowing problems. Mineral oil, if aspirated into the lungs, may cause irritation and even pneumonia.

At age twenty-two, my wife had a cardiac arrest and her brain was deprived of oxygen. She suffered brain damage and was in a coma for weeks. For a long time, she didn't even recognize her two children. We have found comfort focusing on the progress that has been made.

James
Age 26

Some rehabilitation centers have bowel programs to help patients monitor their bowel functions and find appropriate medications to prevent abdominal problems. It is not uncommon to see patients in these programs taking several bowel medications. One goal of a bowel program is to help patients produce a bowel movement every one or two days, at a regular time. To accomplish this, a suppository may be inserted into the rectum just before a meal. Patients then try to have a bowel movement thirty to sixty minutes after the meal. This sequence helps produce a *gastrocolic reflex,* an action in the bowel that occurs when the digestive tract senses new, incoming food. The reflex causes the bowel movement to evacuate any present solid waste.

Diarrhea

Diarrhea describes stool that comes out with a thin, loose consistency or in excessive amounts. Diarrhea may cause cramps because the gut muscles are pushing the stool through at a rate much faster than normal.

Patients who are unable to take nutrition by mouth and are fed by NG tube or stomach tube may have diarrhea. This may happen until the bowel gets used to that form of feeding, especially if the feeding solution is given in a concentrated form and at a high rate. Rather than trying to medicate the diarrhea, the concentration or amount of food may be reduced for a while.

If diarrhea is caused by bacteria, antibiotics will usually clear up the problem. To determine if medication is needed, a stool sample is evaluated for the presence of bacterial toxins.

Odd as it seems, diarrhea might actually be a sign of constipation and impaction higher up in the colon. The trapped stool blocks solid stool as it is produced. Looser stool may run around the obstruction. The patient and nursing staff may only notice diarrhea, a false signal. Medication may only worsen the diarrhea. Abdominal X-rays can help show the stool collection in the colon.

Sexual Problems

A stroke may severely disrupt normal sexual activities. Couples may struggle to regain closeness and intimacy. Sexual activity may be further complicated for patients who suffered a heart attack at the same time as a stroke. The couple may have concerns about the effect of physical exertion on the heart. Individuals should also be aware of high blood pressure and be sure it is under satisfactory control, especially if it contributed to the stroke. Sometimes a partner is afraid that sexual activity may hurt the patient or even trigger another stroke. A doctor can address both general health concerns and the patient's physical readiness for intercourse.

If the stroke has damaged the part of the brain responsible for personality, the change will not likely lead to increased intimacy and closeness. Frustration, agitation, self-pity, depression, and even outward aggression may appear, either due to brain damage or as an emotional response to the stroke. A patient's self-image may deteriorate to the point that he no longer feels sexually attractive. The patient may even feel incapable of love and sexual relations. These emotions tend to keep a partner at a distance.

At the same time, providing the amount of care needed to help a severely affected stroke patient may physically wear out a partner. The partner may lack interest and energy. A lot of courage is usually needed to initiate discussions about sex. If attempts to communicate fail, it may be helpful to contact a rehabilitation psychologist for advice and counseling.

If the stroke has resulted in loss of sensation in the face, limbs, trunk, or sex organs, partners must discover which areas remain sensitive to touch. Paralysis of the limbs may require learning and using different sexual positions. Spasticity may also interfere with sex. For example, spasticity may pull a woman's hips together so tightly that penetration is difficult or impossible.

Language problems may block the ability to communicate the desire for, or the fear of, sex. This can lead to misunderstandings, further increasing a patient's or partner's sense of isolation.

If urinary devices like indwelling catheters are in place, intercourse may be difficult or impossible. One option is to temporarily fold over a catheter inserted into the penis and place a condom over it. If the bladder of a person of either gender requires intermittent use of a catheter, it should be drained before intercourse.

Depression in male stroke patients may be severe enough to cause impotence. Physical causes of impotence may include medications, poor circulation, and diabetes. Sometimes reassurance may be all that is needed. If impotence persists, a patient may need a psychological or urological evaluation. Urologists have new methods to help men regain satisfying sexual relations. For example, urologists may prescribe a medication injected into the penis to cause an erection.

Overall, the quality of the couple's relationship before the stroke is a good predictor of how things will go afterward. The loving and caring attitude that sustains many relationships can help a partner face the challenges of the stroke. Sex is more than intercourse. It encompasses all the tender touches, loving looks, and caring words that bring two people together. Even though certain aspects of sex may change or be altered, some forms of intimate communication will still be available.

7

Other Medical Complications Caused by Strokes

When the effects of a stroke complicate existing physical ailments, a patient's disabilities may increase. A variety of other conditions may affect a patient's recovery from a stroke.

Circulatory Problems

Blood clots, especially those caused by immobility, are of special concern for stroke patients. Through movement, a normal body balances blood circulation and blood clotting. Because many stroke patients are at least partially immobile, blood clots may form, especially in the legs. When a leg is immobile, the blood flow in the leg veins may slow enough to turn to sludge and form clots. Pain, redness, and warmth appear as circulation is impaired.

Onset of these symptoms can be quite sudden and hard to diagnose because stroke patients may experience leg pain for other reasons, such as arthritis. About 30 percent of all stroke patients experience these leg clots, referred to as *deep venous thrombosis (DVT)*. In some rare cases, these clots may travel through a hole in the heart, then into the arteries and on to the brain, causing another stroke.

These clots also have the potential to travel to the right side of the heart and into the lungs. Clot migration into the lungs, called *pulmonary embolus,* occurs in about 10 percent of patients with blood clots. Symptoms such as a rapid heart rate, sudden chest pain, and difficulty breathing may suddenly occur. If a clot is large enough, it may block the flow of blood from the heart to the lungs with deadly results. Pulmonary emboli constitute a medical emergency and must be treated in an intensive care unit, where a patient's changing medical status may be closely monitored. To test for pulmonary emboli, a doctor will order a *ventilation-perfusion scan.* Here, chemicals are injected into the blood and the patient inhales a special gas. If the results show clots have reached the lungs, the doctor will decide whether to anticoagulate the patient.

After my mother's stroke, she was closer to death than life. She made a slow but steady recovery. She continues to touch the lives of those who know her and she lives bravely and with dignity, even though she's changed by a chronic illness.

John
Age 40

Anticoagulation is the use of medicines, often called "blood thinners," to prevent further blood clots. Anticoagulants will not, however, dissolve blood clots already present. The patient is typically given the blood thinner *heparin* through an intravenous line. Later, the patient switches to an oral anticoagulant such as *warfarin* for about three to six months. Not all stroke patients are good candidates for anticoagulation. For example, anticoagulants may worsen problems for a patient who has experienced a stroke due to bleeding in the brain. For these patients, a treatment alternative may be an *inferior vena cava filter*. This device is placed by snaking a tube through a leg vein into the large vein leading to the heart. The device is left there to prevent larger, life-threatening clots from reaching the heart, although smaller ones may still sneak by. Unfortunately, these filters cannot do anything to treat clots that have already traveled to the lungs.

Patients treated with anticoagulants are usually ordered to stay in bed so that blood clots in the legs are not dislodged. Active rehabilitation efforts like dressing, transfers, leg strengthening, and walking are put on hold until it is safe to begin remobilization of the affected leg. Other rehabilitation processes, such as speech therapy and arm strengthening, may still be possible.

Efforts to avoid blood clots may also include prescribing elastic stockings. These special stockings may prevent leg clots by compressing the veins in the legs and encouraging blood movement. Also, inflatable plastic sleeves that alternately pump and then release air may be placed on the foot or the calf to squeeze the veins and help pump blood. There is no perfect protection against clot formation, but these measures can help.

Seizures

Seizures may occur when the brain attempts to transmit electrical charges through the border zone between living tissue and dead tissue caused by a stroke. Roughly 15 percent of stroke patients experience seizures as a result of these interrupted signals. Some evidence suggests that patients who have seizures soon after, or at the time of, a stroke may be at higher risk for developing seizures later on.

Seizures are also referred to as *epilepsy* or *convulsions*. If the number of nerve cells involved is relatively low, a patient may experience a "light" seizure with temporary loss of control and/or shaking of a limb. The patient may also "blank out," staring off into space for several seconds. If the disorganized signal spreads to other areas of the brain, the patient may instead suffer a sudden loss of consciousness as the lips turn blue, breathing becomes difficult, violent shaking racks the body, and bowel or bladder control is lost. This is called a *tonic-clonic seizure* and is also referred to as a *"grand mal"* seizure. Some individuals have sensations that warn when a seizure is about to occur. They have a chance to sit or lie down before they lose consciousness. Seizure patients may be very groggy and confused for several hours after they wake up. They may experience *Todd's paralysis*, limb weakness that can last up to several days. Seizures may mimic initial stroke symptoms, making them difficult to diagnose and differentiate from strokes.

When I was paralyzed, I wasn't sure I wanted to live, but when I began to make progress in recovery, I decided I wanted to get better. Determination is a strong factor. You wonder each day if you're getting better, but you look back and you can see progress.

Tony
Age 74

It is rare for seizures to continue. But if a patient experiences one seizure after another, or if the seizures do not end in a few minutes, the patient may be in *status epilepticus*. This condition is a life-threatening medical emergency because it vastly increases brain metabolism, which in turn uses up the brain's available oxygen and glucose, resulting in more brain damage or even death.

A neurologist may perform *electroencephalograms* (EEGs) to measure electrical impulses in the brain and pinpoint brain damage. Doctors may choose to place patients with abnormal brain waves on medications called anticonvulsants to prevent further seizures. Unfortunately, one side effect of these medications is drowsiness. This can slow rehabilitation progress because patients may not be alert enough to understand instructions, or they may be too tired to fully participate in physical activities.

Once a person experiences a seizure, he may no longer be able to drive a car. Every state in the country has laws governing when people with seizures can drive. A doctor's statement showing the type and severity of the seizure and the prescribed medication must be presented to the licensing authorities. Individuals normally need to be seizure-free for a specified period of time before a department of motor vehicles will consider granting a driver's license.

Pain

Damage to nerve tissue may cause either a loss of sensation or pain. The subcortical brain contains the *thalamus,* a relay center that receives sensory signals from the body and spinal cord and sends new signals to the cortical brain to interpret a stimulus (light/deep touch, hot/cold, vibrations, and so on). Damage to this area may cause *thalamic pain syndrome,* in which the opposite side of the body feels intense, burning pain. Medications may be tried, but this syndrome can be very difficult to treat.

For reasons that remain unclear, the *sympathetic nervous system* may produce pain after a stroke. The sympathetic nervous system is part of the greater involuntary nervous system, which controls those things we do without trying, such as breathing. One theory is that the nerves of the sympathetic nervous system are arranged near those that transmit pain signals in the spinal cord. Some speculate that a "false" relay may develop between these two areas. The result may be *reflex sympathetic dystrophy syndrome (RSD)*. Symptoms in the limbs may include pain, swelling, discoloration, alteration in blood flow, and uncontrolled sweating. Limbs may first turn red and feel hot, then later turn purple and feel cold. The pain can be excruciating. Walking, dressing, and other ADLs may become impossible. The quicker a diagnosis can be made and treatment started, the more successful the outcome. Range-of-motion exercises to stretch the joints and hot/cold contrast baths may help some RSD patients. Others may need medication to break up the influence of the sympathetic nerves. Sometimes, injections into the neck or back may knock out the sympathetic nerves that flow into a limb. In some cases, surgery may be performed, but by the time a patient gets to that stage the chances for a cure are small. Unsuccessful treatment leaves a patient with a limb that is cold, discolored, painful, contracted, and useless.

Musculoskeletal pain is also common after a stroke, caused by muscles either pulling on joints or failing to support them. This can really aggravate existing pain from arthritis or bursitis. For example, a group of four muscles forms the rotator cuff in the shoulder. If the rotator cuff is significantly weakened, the arm is pulled downward by gravity. This *shoulder subluxation* tugs on the tendons and nerves. Slings may provide some measure of support, as they counteract the pull of gravity. Yet some tugging may continue. Even worse, any movement of the shoulder may cause pain or tear the rotator cuff. Musculoskeletal pain is a real barrier to movement and rehabilitation.

Persistent headaches may be another source of pain following a hemorrhage in the brain. These headaches may be as incapacitating as migraines and may make a patient nauseated or sensitive to light. It is important to understand that some of these headaches may last several months and may not respond to pain medications. People with poor bed/wheelchair positioning or trunk/neck muscle weakness may also develop muscle tension headaches, which may be helped by medication and physical therapy. Anxiety and depression may also produce headaches.

Fractures

If a patient is unable to move a limb, over time calcium escapes from the bones. Weakened, brittle bones may break with minimal stress. For stroke patients with limited mobility or impaired balance, even the most seemingly minor falls can result in broken bones. Depending upon the area involved and the severity of the break, a patient may need a cast or an operation.

Edema

Immobility can result in abnormal swelling or fluid buildup, called edema. In a normal body, muscle contractions help "pump" fluid out of the limbs. But when limbs are paralyzed or immobilized, fluid instead collects in the spaces between tissues. If a limb is below the level of the heart, gravity will pull fluid into the limb. This is why many people who develop edema may experience very little swelling in the morning but collect a lot of fluid by the end of the day.

Edema can be treated in a variety of ways. *Diuretic medications*, commonly called "water pills," may help rid the body of extra fluid. Compressive stockings or elastic wraps may put pressure on the capillary beds to prevent fluid from resting in the tissues. If swelling is severe—even to the point of making the skin stretch so much that it breaks open—a mechanical edema pump may be used. An edema pump uses external pressure to force fluid out of the tissues and back into circulation. Edema in the loose skin at the back of the hands may affect the ability of the fingers to bend and grip, resulting in *contractures*. Wearing an elastic glove, elevating the arm on foam wedges and placing the hands on a lap board may help drain fluid. Edema pumps for the arms may also be prescribed. Therapists may apply compression wraps to each finger and massage them to encourage fluid mobility.

Decubitus Ulcers

Decubitus ulcers, also called bedsores, usually form as the result of prolonged pressure on the skin. Normally, the sensation of touch prompts us to move around when we sit or lie down, relieving the pressure. Stroke patients may lose this ability, or they may not have the strength or coordination to shift away from the pressure. Decubitus ulcers typically form over bony areas such as the heels, ankle bones, and several areas around the pelvis.

Elderly stroke patients are at high risk of developing decubitus ulcers since they may have lost skin elasticity as well as some of the fat underneath their skin. This makes their skin more fragile. Even pulling off an adhesive bandage may tear the top layer of their skin and cause bleeding. Likewise, the simple act of raising the head of a hospital bed may cause a patient to slide down. The friction against the backside may contribute to the development of skin sores.

Doctors grade the amount of damage to the skin by the appearance of skin redness or the depth of skin breakdown. Treatment is based upon the severity of the wound.

Table 2. Decubitus Ulcer Grades

Grade 1	Redness does not blanch to finger pressure and may not break down. Usually treated conservatively.
Grade 2	Erosion down to the fat under the skin. This does not blanch to finger pressure. May be treated conservatively or with a skin graft.
Grade 3	Erosion down to the level of muscle. Requires surgical correction.
Grade 4	Erosion down to the level of bone. Requires surgical correction.

The first two decubitus ulcer grades include the most superficial breakdowns that may extend into the fat layer. Removing pressure points is the first step toward healing and prevention of decubitus ulcers. If the surface area is large or infected, surgery may be required to clean up dead tissue. The patient may also require a *split thickness skin graft,* in which skin from another area is used to cover an open wound. The graft will promote faster healing. If the wound is deep enough to reach muscle tissue or bone, it will not heal well without an operation like a *muscle rotation flap,* in which muscle and skin from an adjoining area are rotated over a wound.

Special mattresses or padded coverings around the feet may help prevent skin ulcers. Wheelchair cushions may help prevent sores on the buttocks caused by sitting too long in one position. Even with proper precautions, there is no guarantee that skin will not break down. Stroke patients with diabetes may have an even more difficult time feeling the effects of pressure against the skin because the disease may damage the small nerves of the hands and especially the legs. Unaware of cuts and burns, their wounds may become infected. A diabetic's metabolism doesn't promote normal healing.

Patients with leg numbness are at higher risk of developing skin sores because they may not feel pressure, may not have the strength to reposition themselves, or may not have the language ability to tell others that they feel pain from pressure against the skin. Patients who are poorly nourished or have a low red blood cell count *(anemia)* may be more prone to skin sores and may heal more slowly. Proper nutrition includes proteins to provide the building blocks for healing wounds. Rarely, a blood transfusion is used to increase the red blood cell count and to encourage the skin to heal.

In recent years, hospitals have developed specialty centers to provide care for difficult wounds and skin damage. One promising technique sometimes used by wound centers is *platelet-derived growth factor*. Here, special parts of the patient's own blood are cultivated and then applied to the wound to promote healing.

Part III

Recovery and Rehabilitation

8

Recovery: What to Expect

"How much recovery can we expect?" This is usually the first question asked by stroke survivors and their loved ones. Unfortunately, medical caregivers cannot absolutely predict the outcome of the rehabilitation process. The best they can do is make estimates based on clinical studies and expertise, taking into account the patient's trend of improvement.

Stroke Severity

Overall, successful recovery from a stroke depends on the extent of damage to brain tissue and the location of the damage in the brain. Many of the brain's functions seem to be localized in specific regions. Therefore, the injury will affect the body functions governed by a particular region. For example, a marble-sized area of damage in the upper cortical levels of the brain may cause weakness in the hand. Yet the same sized damage in the brain stem may result in worse symptoms such as paralysis of an arm and a leg because so many more nerves funnel into this area. Blockages of the brain's larger blood vessels, caused by heavy bleeding into the skull cavity, usually causes irreparable damage. Severe brain damage may result in death.

Patients who have other diseases that might worsen during the rehabilitation process (*comorbidity*) may not be good candidates for therapy. This is particularly true of elderly stroke patients. Likewise, comatose patients or those supported by high-tech equipment are not ready for rehabilitation, although some bedside therapies may be appropriate.

When my stroke hit, I felt numb all over. I was scared and confused. I forgot my family's names. I am glad for the aggressive rehabilitation I've had; it keeps my mind focused on what I need to do to get better.

Ken
Age 53

Neurological Recovery

Neurological recovery is a medical term used to describe the healing of brain tissue. The brain forms an extremely complex web of nerve tissue that controls the body through electrical impulses, much like the fuse box in a house controls electricity leading to various circuits, lights, and outlets. Assume for a moment that lightning strikes the house. It may be difficult to determine which circuits were affected. It may be even harder to determine if appliances were damaged. The brain is millions of times more complex than house wiring. Therefore, it is difficult to say with precision how much neurological damage might have resulted from a stroke.

Neurological recovery will also depend on the extent of *unmasking* that occurs. In this process, undamaged brain tissue assumes some of the functions of the dead tissue. The potential of living nerves is "unmasked," or opened up, to help with recovery. Nerves may also heal by *sprouting*. When a nerve connection is lost, nerve cells may send out new "sprouts" in search of connections. However, sprouts may not be able to reestablish old connections if large parts of the brain are damaged or if sprouts become trapped in scar tissue.

Brain functions may also improve once swelling from a stroke diminishes. Just as a finger swells with inflammatory fluid after it is crushed, the brain swells inside the skull when it is damaged by a stroke. Nerves do not function well under this type of pressure. Swelling and pressure inside the head usually subside within days or weeks, restoring some nerve functions. If the swelling doesn't subside, a patient may not survive.

Functional Recovery

Functional recovery describes a patient's ability to regain activities of daily living—ADLs. Functional recovery is affected by both neurological recovery and rehabilitation.

The patient's age is also a factor in recovery. Generally, chances of recovery decrease with increasing age. This is partially due to the brain's healing process—plasticity—the ability of the remaining healthy brain to take over the functions of the damaged brain. As we age, this process becomes less effective.

Another factor in recovery is how soon rehabilitation begins after a stroke. The goal is to have patients begin therapy as soon as possible. Those who begin therapy right away, rather than weeks or months later, will make more progress.

Finally, functional recovery is also influenced by positive attitudes—both a patient's and those of family members. Noted psychologist William James teaches that attitude is the most important determinant to success. We may all apply his teachings to stroke recovery. If the patient is unable to develop a positive attitude as a result of brain damage, it is important that friends and family create a supportive, positive environment. "Problems" viewed instead as "challenges" are more easily overcome. Such gentle shifts in thinking can be most helpful. The key to rehabilitation is to use whatever works.

It is also important that family and friends do as much as possible to educate themselves about stroke and recovery. Information may be gleaned from a variety of sources—the health-care team, educational books and videos, and stroke education classes.

As social workers, we help resolve financial concerns, provide emotional support, help coordinate services, help with discharge planning, and direct families to appropriate resources.

Roghie, 60
Case Manager

Medical Factors Affecting Recovery

Anemia

Anemia, a low number of red blood cells, limits the ability of the blood to carry oxygen to the brain. This in turn limits a patient's physical abilities since exercise consumes more oxygen than immobility. Most therapeutic functional rehabilitation involves physical exertion.

Arthritis

Moderate to severe *arthritis,* inflammation of the joint tissue, may cause enough pain to prevent patients from ever again being able to walk. Arthritic patients may not be able to tolerate the weight of standing, even if supporting themselves with canes or walkers. Other painful joints may interfere with activities like dressing, grooming, and transfers.

Heart Disease

Severe heart problems may prevent any rehabilitation efforts. A fair number of stroke patients have heart attacks in addition to a stroke, making heart damage an immediate concern. Doctors use their best judgment when deciding if a patient's heart is strong enough to handle therapeutic exercise.

Angina, chest pain due to a lack of oxygen to the heart, may become so painful that one cannot exercise. Patients with angina may even suffer heart attacks when they exert themselves. Medical conditions in which the heart's pumping function is marginal, as in congestive heart failure, may not permit patients to perform enough physical work to participate in therapies.

Atrial fibrillation (AF) is a condition in which irregular heartbeats can allow blood to sludge within the heart and form clots. AF adds two complicating factors to the rehabilitation process. First, it may increase the possibility of further strokes from emboli. Second, the blood-pumping ability of the heart is reduced by 10 to 15 percent, further depriving the body of oxygen and limiting exercise tolerance.

If you have a large family, it's best to have one family representative relay information between the hospital staff and other family members. When people are dealing with a crisis, they may not absorb everything you tell them, so repetition is important.

Vivian, 57
Case Manager

Lung Disease

Many people who have strokes are longtime smokers. Smoking can result in lung diseases such as asthma and emphysema. Any type of lung disease limits the amount of oxygen that enters the body, thus limiting a person's ability to exercise. Smokers and others with chronic lung diseases usually do not exercise much. Therefore, they are often in poor physical condition when they have a stroke.

Skin Problems

In the previous chapter, we examined how bed sores can eventually result from stroke. Similarly, if skin breakdown is already a problem, it is will impair recovery efforts. Patients with these problems are not good candidates for rehabilitation because any movement may stretch and tear their skin. Although these people cannot usually participate in activities involving walking or sitting, they may be able to rebuild strength by participating in limited activities.

There is an extraordinary healing power in love. I never underestimate the healing power of a kind word of encouragement, a smile, a gentle touch, or a shoulder to cry on. Patients need to be told that they will make it and that they are not alone.
Jean, 41
Hospital Supervisor

Low Endurance

Bed rest can be debilitating. One week of strict bed rest can result in up to a 15 percent loss of muscle strength and endurance. These problems get worse the longer a patient is in bed. Regaining strength takes at least twice as long as it did to lose, even if no complicating medical problems exist. This deconditioning, or *immobilization syndrome*, significantly prolongs the remobilization process.

Impaired Eyesight, Hearing, and Touch

Vision and hearing problems may interfere with the ability to communicate and relearn ADLs. If a patient can no longer understand speech, therapists may need to use hand signals to communicate. Progress becomes quite difficult if the patient can neither see the gestures nor hear well enough to understand spoken instructions.

Diabetes

Diabetes may cause deterioration of the small vessels of the eyes. This leads to poor vision, even blindness. It can also result in a stroke. Diabetes may damage the small nerves in the hands, legs, and feet, making limbs numb. This numbness may affect activities from dressing to walking and may make diabetics prone to injuries that they can't feel. If these injuries become infected, amputation can result, further hampering rehabilitation.

Malnutrition

Studies have shown that people who are malnourished tend to need extended hospital stays and also may have lower functional outcomes. Although hospital dietitians can design menus to try to overcome this problem, stroke patients with dysphagia—difficulty swallowing—may have trouble consuming adequate quantities of food.

> *After stroke, life goes on and can be good again. Many have told me they experience a change in life's priorities. People, especially family, become much more important. Joy is found in things previously taken for granted.*
>
> *Pat, 47*
> *Rehabilitation*
> *Counselor*

Mortality Rates

Unfortunately, most people who have had one stroke are statistically more likely to have more strokes, although this certainly does not happen to everyone. If there are additional strokes, it may take quite some time before they happen. Regardless of the type of stroke, the larger the area of the brain deprived of blood and oxygen, the worse the outcome and the higher the chance of death. About 56 percent of people who suffer bleeding into the brain, an intracerebral hemorrhage, die within the first month. The pressure of trapped blood and swelling brain tissue built up inside the bony skull results in death for up to 82 percent of these patients within the first week. This pressure, called *mass effect,* pushes the brain away, forcing it down toward the hole in the base of the skull where the brain and spinal cord meet. Compressed into this narrowed opening, the vital functions of the brain stem stop and the patient dies.

Studies have shown that people who suffer subarachnoid hemorrhages, bleeding into the space around the brain, usually die within three months if the critical volume of blood leakage exceeds twenty milliliters, an amount equivalent to four teaspoonfuls of fluid. About 50 percent of people with subarachnoid hemorrhages die as a result of a first stroke. The chance of recurrent bleeding is about 3.5 percent each year if the subarachnoid hemorrhage is not treated with surgery. If a second bleeding episode occurs, the chance of death is around 67 percent. Patients with intraventricular hemorrhages, where bleeding spreads into the deep cavities of the brain, are better able to survive. However, survivors of subarachnoid hemorrhages tend to recover better than those with intraventricular hemorrhages.

9

Rehabilitation

Rehabilitation is the process by which health-care providers systematically work to help patients restore as many mental and physical functions as possible. However, a patient's medical stability and endurance are the first considerations in determining readiness for rehabilitation. Most rehabilitation centers set up carefully tailored programs for those patients who are ready for rehabilitation. Readiness also requires motivation on the part of the patient. At this point, motivation is the key.

Levels of Care

Rehabilitation goals are constantly assessed to determine where patients fit in the spectrum of care. The most intense level of rehabilitation care is *acute care* delivered in the hospital. At this level, patients are actively involved daily in any combination of physical therapy, occupational therapy, and speech therapy for three hours a day, five days a week. Patients who can't meet the strength and endurance criteria may best be served at a lower level of medical care, such as that offered by a subacute rehabilitation unit or a skilled care unit. Here, they can build endurance until they are ready to begin more demanding therapy. *Subacute rehabilitation* usually accommodates people who need about two hours of therapy per day. *Skilled care* is for patients who may be able to handle one therapy per day but who also have other skilled nursing needs. Patients who have reached a plateau but who are still not able to go home may find *nursing home care* an alternative. Some nursing homes may offer physical, occupational, and speech therapy to help patients continue to make progress toward eventually returning home.

My husband's therapy began soon after his stroke. At first, he needed two people to help him walk. After one month, only one therapist was needed. Now, he can get in and out of a chair with only a little help.

Marie
Age 79

Levels of Assistance

A *level of assistance* refers to the amount of help needed to perform self-care activities or ADLs. The rehabilitation team evaluates each patient's assistance levels to determine how much assistance will be needed once the patient returns home.

A patient at the *dependent assist level* needs caregivers providing all ADLs. For example, the patient may need the help of several nurses to move from a bed to a wheelchair.

Maximum assist level describes someone who needs 75 percent of ADLs performed by a caregiver. A patient at this level typically needs a caregiver to do most of the work during an activity such as standing to dress.

A patient able to perform about half the ADLs is ranked at the *moderate assist level.* At this point, some patients are able to go home successfully if someone there is available to help them.

Minimal assist is the level at which a patient needs about 25 percent help for ADLs. *Contact guard assist* is the level at which some "hands-on" help is provided for activities during which a person could be injured by falling, such as walking. A person who has recovered quite well but still has minor balance or safety risks is rated at the *standby assist level*. Finally, if a patient can perform a specific task alone, he is considered *independent* in that skill.

Monitoring Progress

On a regular basis, a rehabilitation team will measure and score a patient's ability to perform a variety of activities like walking, transferring, speaking, and going to the bathroom. The scores will reflect how dependent or independent the patient is in each area. The trends in progress help determine the length of the patient's stay in a rehabilitation unit. The patient may continue to stay as scores improve. Once scores do not change, the patient may be ready for discharge. However, even if scores level off and the patient is discharged, he may still strive for improvement. Although these scores may not be an exact predictor of recovery to come, they may give friends and families some idea of how much improvement they may expect in the future.

Take everything one day at a time. Realize early on that recovery takes time and patience. If you give up, your progress will go much slower or will stop.

Linda
Age 47

Rehabilitation Professionals

During rehabilitation, a patient will meet a number of rehabilitation professionals, all of whom are usually part of a team. Usually a medical doctor called a *physiatrist*, who specializes in rehabilitation, directs the team effort. A number of other professionals—rehabilitation nurses, physical therapists, occupational therapists, speech pathologists, rehabilitation psychologists, social workers, therapeutic recreation specialists, orthotists, and prosthotists—all add their expertise to the effort. Hospital chaplains and other physicians may also join the rehabilitation team.

Nurses

Rehabilitation nurses specialize in taking care of stroke patients going through rehabilitation. They provide direct medical care—giving medications, assisting with feeding, providing bladder and bowel care. They also play a vital role in rehabilitation, communicating information to physicians and other team members. Since they spend more time with patients than do other team members, nurses are in a unique position to observe and assess patients. Nurses are also the ones who often educate patients and their families and friends about medical care.

Physical Therapists

Physical therapists (PTs) focus on maximizing one's mobility and independence. Always with safety in mind, they help patients improve walking, balance, strength, leg coordination and range of joint motion. Learning to walk again is usually a rigorous challenge. How do PTs approach this task?

PTs may have patients begin the walking process using parallel bars, similar to those used by gymnasts. A *gait belt* is snugged around the waist or under the arms to help safely guide patients as they shift their weight and take their first steps. Then, depending on improvement, walking equipment may be introduced, including an *elevated walker,* a *hemi-cane* (a large, four-legged device), or other types of walkers, canes, or crutches. To help overcome balance problems and weakness, PTs may help patients with a variety of exercises, including those done on mats. Other therapies often directed by PTs include upper and lower limb cycles and weights to build strength and endurance.

Occupational Therapists

Occupational therapists (*OTs*) focus on patients' regaining the ability to do basic daily activities—dressing, grooming, and using the toilet. OTs show patients how to use many types of adaptive equipment—wheelchairs, home bath benches, special eating utensils, and long-handled doorknobs. OTs may visit patients' homes to identify any needs for adaptive equipment. Normally, equipment is ordered and installed before hospital discharge. It is best if a patient can visit with an OT during a home assessment to discuss individual needs and possible obstacles such as narrow doorways, thick carpets, or small bathrooms.

> *It is important for nurses to give patients as much emotional support as possible. Nurses can also anticipate the needs of patients' communication problems; speak slowly, in short sentences for the aphasic patient.*
>
> *Mary, 33*
> *RN*

OTs also help patients learn to make transfers. The word *transfer* is used a lot during the rehabilitation process. The term refers to the process of moving from one surface to another. Typical transfers done in the course of a hospital day include bed to wheelchair, wheelchair to toilet, wheelchair to mat, and wheelchair to shower chair.

Speech Pathologists

Speech pathologists help restore language skills and help patients learn other ways to communicate, if necessary. Speech pathologists also work with patients who may need swallowing therapy as a result of dysphagia.

Neuropsychologists

Emotional recovery from a stroke is challenging, to say the least. Most comprehensive rehabilitation centers have psychologists available to help patients adjust to new circumstances, especially if a stroke has affected the part of the brain that regulates personality.

Counseling can help patients develop balance in their lives. Psychologists help patients direct their energy toward new goals—returning home and taking the best possible care of themselves.

Social Workers

Medical *social workers* (also called *hospital case managers*) are actually an "advance team" working to make sure that patients have the skills and services they need once they leave the health-care environment. The medical social worker's goal, from day one, is to help patients plan for discharge from the hospital. For example, if a patient needs to go to a nursing home, the social worker can help find the most suitable, affordable, and convenient place available. Many nursing homes have a long waiting list. Social workers can help cut through the red tape.

Medical social workers often play an important role in helping families identify financial resources to pay for hospital stays and ongoing expenses. Social workers will be aware of

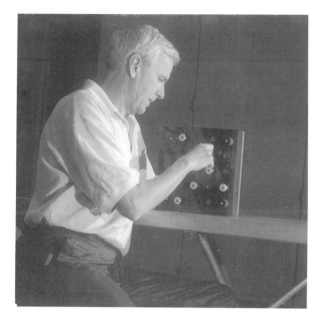

Recovery requires patience, persistence, and repetition. Repeating these peg board exercises helps improve coordination. Developing a coordinated pattern of muscle motion may require thousands, even millions, of repetitions.

The goal of speech therapy is to improve speaking ability as well as other complex communication skills. Here, the patient is relearning to associate written words with specific objects.

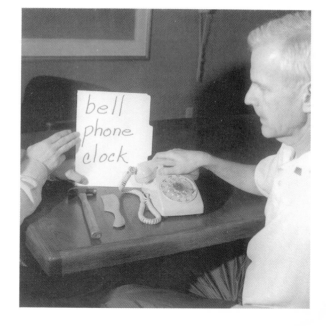

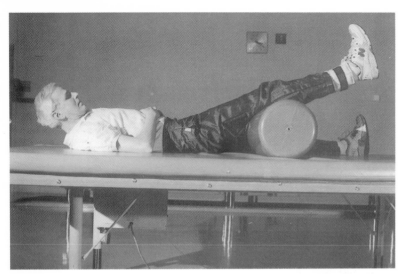

Guided therapeutic exercises on
the mats strengthen muscles
and build coordination. Above, the
patient uses a tubular bolster under the
leg, which allows motion to occur in
isolated muscles.

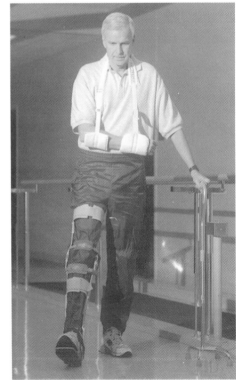

Braces are used to help build strength,
balance, and coordination in walking.
Here, a long-leg brace and a 4-pronged
cane help the patient strive for higher
levels of mobility.

An arm support sling helps build strength and coordination in the arm. The sling eliminates the effects of gravity, making it easier to practice movements.

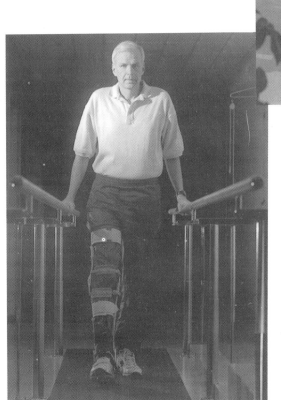

In physical therapy, parallel bars provide support and balance for learning to walk again. Early on, use of the bars helps therapists assess walking ability.

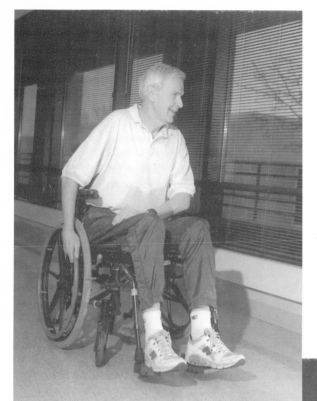

For some patients, wheelchairs offer mobility. Use of a wheelchair also strengthens muscles in the arms and upper body. Wheelchairs can be modified to best fit the patients' needs.

This driving simulator evaluates the ability to drive safely. The simulator tests judgment, reaction time, and the ability to sequence activities. The coordination of vision with arm and leg movement is also measured.

help available through various social and governmental agencies, and they can speed much of the paperwork, which can range from obtaining a handicapped parking permit to filling out Medicaid applications. These services can be most helpful to those coping with both the physical and emotional consequences of stroke.

Note that patients and families often confuse medical social workers, employed by a hospital, with *case managers* who work for insurance companies. The insurance case manager's goal is to analyze the cost to the insurance company and to make sure that costly, "unnecessary" care is not provided.

Therapeutic Recreation Specialists

These *recreation specialists* strive to provide recreation—a break from the concentration required for medical therapies. Having fun is important to a balanced life. And, patients may need to learn new activities or modify the types of activities they previously enjoyed. A patient whose stroke has affected a dominant arm might strengthen the nondominant arm by working on crafts and writing skills. Other recreation therapies might include painting or playing cards and board games. Later, patients may be involved in community reentry activities, in which they take field trips, go shopping, or go to the bank.

Patients seem to make the most progress when they have a means to cope. Loved ones can provide the support that is so essential in recovery.
Sharon, 29
Physical Therapist

An important part of therapeutic recreation is *socialization*, in which patients join in planned activities that provide them an opportunity to interact with others with disabilities. The goal is to lessen their feelings of isolation and to make them aware that they are not the only ones to face the challenges of a stroke. Sometimes, speaking to other patients in similar situations helps reduce their fears. This may foster a sense of mutual encouragement and lead to friendships that extend past the hospital stay.

A popular program offered by some rehabilitation centers is pet therapy. Animals, usually dogs and cats, are brought in to visit the patients. Interacting with animals can help patients relieve stress and depression and even tap unrealized speech potential.

Pet therapy can be very motivating. As one patient told me, "Dogs have an amazing knowledge of what each patient needs. Animals seem to distance patients from a consuming sense of loss."
Kris, 40
Recreational Therapist

Orthotists and Prosthotists

Orthotists are specialists who make braces and splints for limbs. Sometimes a brace is needed to better position a limb or to help compensate for weakness caused by a stroke. Many patients will need leg support to make walking possible again. Leg braces can be custom-made by the orthotist to improve balance, safety, and walking efficiency. *Prosthotists* make and adjust artificial limbs. The loss of limbs, through amputation, may occur in stroke patients who are diabetics or who have extremely poor circulation in the legs.

Hospital Chaplains

Commonly, spiritual support is provided by *hospital chaplains.*They visit patients on a regular basis and are on call in times of crisis. They provide spiritual counsel, advice, and prayer that many people find comforting. Chaplains help calm fears by putting stroke disabilities in a spiritual context.

86

Other Physicians

People affected by stroke often have complex diseases and medical needs best addressed by physician specialists. *Internal medicine* and *family practice physicians* provide care for ongoing medical conditions like diabetes and blood pressure. *Cardiologists* and *pulmonologists* specialize in heart and lung problems. *Urologists* evaluate bladder problems. *Psychiatrists* may provide medication and counseling for patients with depression or behavioral problems. Visual problems are assessed by *ophthalmologists. Plastic surgeons* may provide wound care management.

10

Aftercare

Plans for the return home begin the day a stroke patient enters the hospital. The term *aftercare* encompasses all the processes involved in discharging a patient from the hospital and arranging for a comfortable environment. The first consideration is where the patient will be living—in a facility, at home, or in a relative's home. Aftercare plans are customized to the needs of the patient.

Rehabilitation case managers try to make it possible for patients to continue making progress in the rehabilitation effort. Case managers may set up handicapped transportation, acquire equipment, and schedule subsequent therapies, lab tests, and follow-up visits with physicians. They may also act as intermediaries between the patient/family and insurance companies to determine what moneys are available to help pay for aftercare needs.

The medical team will decide whether the patient will be able to travel to the hospital, rehabilitation center, or other location for therapy services or whether these will need to be provided in the home. Home health-care agencies can provide nursing, therapies, and treatments to patients who are homebound or extremely disabled. Outpatient visits to the hospital or rehabilitation center are preferred if more than one therapist is needed, or if specialized equipment, only available at a rehabilitation hospital, is required.

Therapists and doctors will see that appropriate therapies are provided. Usually, once the patient has reached a plateau or has achieved his goals, formal therapy is discontinued. This does not mean, however, that the patient has achieved full potential.

Patients may continue to improve themselves mentally and physically after formal therapies have ended by performing a program of exercises, either alone or with the help of friends and family. Therapists and doctors will be available to offer suggestions and to help determine when these activities have helped the patient reach full potential.

Safety at Home

To plan for a patient's discharge from the hospital to home, everyday skills must be reevaluated. Even the most common activities may become problematic after a stroke. For example, is the patient ready to cook over a hot stove or handle sharp knives in the kitchen?

Other concerns include throw rugs, which can be hazardous for patients who have trouble with balance or eyesight. Stairs can be a problem, especially for those with hemiplegia. Loss of driving skills usually is the most crushing aftereffect of a stroke for many people. Occupational and physical therapists can address the functions needed to resume living at home.

Respite Care

Taking care of a handicapped patient, no matter how loved, can become a heavy burden. Temporary assistance in the care of elderly or disabled individuals is known as *respite care*. It is designed to give caregivers a break from the daily routines associated with long-term disability that can cause physical and emotional burnout. Without relief, the pressure of full-time caregiving may destroy family relationships and personal goals.

After my stroke, I kept asking, "Why me?" Then in therapy I saw others worse off. I began to realize I was pretty lucky. During my first eighteen months of recovery I didn't feel like myself. Even when I returned home, everything was a chore, but I kept trying.

Joan
Age 59

Even the strongest and most loving people need a break from the day-to-day responsibilities of caring for another. Long before this type of strain begins to take its toll, respite care should be discussed with both the patient's doctors and case manager. They know about home-care alternatives and agencies that specialize in respite care. Some communities have day hospital programs that enable the stroke patient to develop a social life. These programs may also offer some level of medical supervision or may facilitate visits by occupational and physical therapists. As an alternative, families and friends may also take turns giving each other time off.

Transportation

Transportation needs may change for a person now coping with disability. For those who have been given permission to drive, they may be aided by any number of adaptive devices—special knobs and pedals—can be installed to make driving easier and safer.

However, for patients who are not ready to drive, it could be extremely dangerous for them to do so. For example, someone with a visual field cut may not see oncoming traffic. The results could be deadly. Losing the ability to drive can be most depressing for those accustomed to driving. This is a time for families and friends to offer extra emotional support and, in some cases, make sure car keys are not accessible.

Still other individuals may find themselves needing special transportation. Perhaps medical equipment will not fit into a standard car, or getting in and out of the car is difficult. There are numerous accommodating modes of transportation. These may include mass transportation systems designed to hold wheelchairs, specially adapted conversion vans, and cars retrofitted for medical equipment. Taxi services for people with disabilities may be available. Doctors may need to complete special forms to document disability and to authorize special transportation and handicapped parking privileges.

> *To assist in driving, we can get all kinds of adaptive equipment----special turn knobs, left foot gas pedal, hand controls, special mirrors. If it is safe for you to drive, but you have some physical weakness, we can help you drive again.*
>
> *Rick, 35*
> *OT/Driving Instructor*

Transportation services vary considerably from one community to another. Thanks to the Americans with Disabilities Act (ADA), communities that offer transportation systems are required to accommodate the needs of the physically challenged traveler. Some transportation services may require reservations up to one week in advance. Others may be able to pick up passengers from the curb but not from the door. An increasing number of companies are entering the field of assisted transportation as the average age of our population increases.

Despite the options available, transportation may still be a problem due to cost or the need for a traveling companion to assist with transfers. Public and accessible transportation may also be exceptionally difficult in rural areas, where it is often most needed. Case managers and physicians may be able to schedule home health-agency visits for rehabilitation and may know of hospitals, senior centers, or churches that offer voluntary or low-cost transportation.

One of the toughest things was dealing with the loss of independence, especially not being able to drive. The desire to drive again made me focus on hard work in therapy.
Dorothy
Age 74

Employment

Returning to the workplace may not be a priority for all stroke patients. However, for younger patients, returning to work may be a critical issue. Not surprisingly, scientific studies indicate that young people with the fewest functional deficits are the most likely to be successful in returning to the workforce. Patients, particularly those with right hemisphere strokes, who have jobs that don't require a lot of physical movement, tend to return to the workforce more easily; they are left with residual weakness that lends itself to adaptive resources. The same is not true for workers whose jobs depend on physical skill. In these cases, evaluations by physicians, neuropsychologists, and vocational counselors will help determine which patients are able to go back to work.

Therapists can give measurable estimates of physical and cognitive abilities. If a work release is granted, stroke patients still need to be aware that anxiety, depression, frustration, and a sense of being overwhelmed by the work environment are still possible. Members of the rehabilitation care team may visit the workplace to check for potential safety problems and work environment challenges, as well as make other suggestions for a smoother transition into the workplace.

Durable Medical Equipment

As a patient gets ready to leave the hospital, the physician, physical therapist, and occupational therapist determine what types of equipment will be needed to help with ADLs at home. Equipment designed for long-term use is called *durable medical equipment* (*DME*). These items can be most helpful but can be very expensive. Because patients may regain functional skills over time, it may be worth renting durable medical equipment rather than buying it. The rehabilitation team may take quite a while to experiment with different devices before they find the best equipment for each patient. As a general guideline, do not purchase any durable medical item until it has been discussed with the appropriate professional.

Sometimes it may not be possible for the right equipment to be acquired until after discharge. Shorter hospital stays often mean having less lead time to make arrangements for equipment and home modifications before a patient is discharged. This frustration is shared by patients, loved ones, and health-care workers alike.

Since insurance, Medicare, and Medicaid coverage constantly changes, it is sometimes impossible to guess what equipment and medical expenses these plans might reimburse. Be sure to ask therapists, medical case managers, insurance case managers, and government representatives specifically what will or won't be covered before a service or piece of equipment is provided.

Braces and Walking Devices

A brace is also known as an *orthosis*. The most common leg brace used after a stroke is an *ankle-foot orthosis (AFO)*. This L-shaped leg brace is available in two types. The first is a double-upright AFO built into a shoe with two long calf bars and a tie band at the upper calf. A mechanical joint is placed near the patient's ankle joint. The ankle joint may be mobile or stationary to accommodate and control ankle and knee motion. The other kind of AFO is made of polypropylene plastic. It has the advantage of being more cosmetic, of lighter weight, and transferable between different shoes if heel heights are the same. It may also have a moving or rigid ankle joint. There is also a type of spring-steel brace for people who don't need a lot of extra support. It attaches to a shoe.

An orthotist will see that all braces are selected or custom-made to provide the best comfort, fit, and ankle/knee control. Use of a physical therapy department's various "stock" AFOs will help determine whether a patient needs a custom-made brace. Arm and leg braces are often prescribed early in the hospital stay if a patient shows a pattern of complete hemiplegia. Some patients recover well enough and fast enough that an expensive or bulky brace is unnecessary. Others may progress to a lighter brace. Physicians and therapists may wait weeks or months to formalize a prescription for expensive braces while assessing a patient's improvement. The final prescription for braces may be finalized after several follow-up clinic visits.

Some patients have knee instability and may fall while walking. Control may be achieved by altering the angle of the ankle joint in the brace. The foot portion of an AFO can tilt the foot down, providing a force against the leg to keep the knee supported in extension. Setting an AFO at a slightly upward angle causes the knee to bend, helping people whose knees tend to overextend backward. Braces like these help with safety by passively lifting the foot during walking to prevent foot-drop. *Foot-drop* happens when the foot drops down toward the ground, or drags, making walking difficult and unsafe. Braces also help decrease the amount of energy it takes to walk. For those people who do not find braces too heavy to use, braces make the difference between walking and being confined to a wheelchair.

> *When I first began walking, the therapist tried a leg brace, but it didn't hold my foot well. Then I tried a custom-made brace. It was easier to put on and more comfortable and made my walking more stable.*
>
> *Arnold*
> *Age 79*

Braces may also help people who lack knee mobility. Use of a knee-ankle-foot orthosis that comes up over the knee may provide enough stability. The trade-off of this type of support is the increased weight and related energy needed to walk compared to using an AFO.

The usual progression of gait and walking devices is as follows: parallel bars, wheeled walker, regular walker, quad cane (one with four feet to improve balance), single-point cane, and hopefully, independent ambulation. Depending upon their initial walking ability, patients may start out using any of these devices. It is not uncommon for a person who has had a stroke to always need some sort of walking device for mobility and safety.

The final prescription for walking aids and braces is usually done close to discharge. Factors involved in prescribing the appropriate device include strength, balance, safety, coordination, ability to sequence activities, visual loss, and the cognitive ability to use the device.

Wheelchairs and Cushions

Occupational therapists usually decide upon the best wheelchair and cushion for each patient. Virtually every component on a wheelchair can be customized. Occupational therapists keep catalogues listing the options. For example, tires may be air-filled or solid rubber. Swing-away foot rests may help with safety during transfers. A brake-extension handle may mean greater independence and improved quality of life for a patient who depends upon using a wheelchair as the main mode of mobility. A good seat cushion may reduce the development of decubitus ulcers on the buttocks of people who spend entire days sitting in a wheelchair. Like all equipment, however, the cushion must be used correctly and consistently to be effective.

Beds and Mattresses

Occasionally, recovering stroke patients will need a hospital bed or special mattress at home to ensure safe transfers, to reduce pressure on fragile skin, or to help change body positions. Hospital beds come in electric and semi-electric models.

Overhead trapezes attached to the bed may help patients position themselves in bed to prevent skin sores and to assist in transfers to and from the bed. Beds that can be raised and lowered in height make transfers much easier, especially from a low wheelchair to the bed.

Special, soft mattresses, used to prevent skin breakdown, may make transfers difficult. The soft bed won't provide as much support to a sitting person as will a normal, firm mattress. These soft mattresses may also be taller than a normal mattress, increasing the difficulty with transfers. Some occupational therapy departments have beds of different heights available to try out before a bed is purchased.

The patient's physician and occupational therapist can determine if a special bed or mattress is necessary. Not everyone needs these devices. Medicare, Medicaid, and most insurance companies will limit coverage of these items and will not pay for them if they are not prescribed.

My main obstacle was making transfers into the wheelchair—I needed two people to help me. But I overcame it once I started therapies. I learned to walk again. I tried to work hard in therapy; each day brought new rewards.

Leone
Age 71

Home Adaptability Devices

Home modifications may add to a stroke patient's quality of life, convenience, and safety. Occupational therapists are often ingenious when it comes to home modifications for the disabled. Before discharge, if possible, it is best for a therapist to visit the patient's home to identify and evaluate barriers and recommend changes. The popular term "handicapped accessible" means that people who have difficulty walking or who use a wheelchair may safely enter a building because it has been modified to handle their needs. Nowhere is accessibility more important than at home. Occupational therapists can point out many potential problems, especially safety issues.

Most patients with mobility problems have difficulty entering their homes. Most homes have steps leading to the entrances. Sturdy handrails on each side of the steps will be helpful for people who can negotiate them. Ramps need to be installed to accommodate people using wheelchairs. For a person to independently move a wheelchair up and down a ramp, the ramp should extend horizontally one foot for every one inch in vertical rise. For example, a ramp needs to be thirty feet long to replace five steps with a six-inch rise from each step. Usually, at least one turn will be built into the ramp. Placement of a ramp may be functional but not cosmetic. A ramp may be constructed of wood or have cement foundations. Before a ramp is installed, homeowners should first estimate how long it may be needed. If a patient is recovering fairly rapidly, building a ramp may not be worth the expense. If it appears that the stroke patient is going to need a ramp for years, a quality ramp will be a good investment. Therapists may be able to provide a list of contractors willing to provide cost estimates and design suggestions for ramp construction.

> *Some days in therapy will go more smoothly than others, but try to maintain a positive attitude and focus on what you can do. Improvement comes in small steps. View them as building blocks toward your goal.*
> *Julie, 35*
> *Occupational Therapist*

Once inside the home, doorways, hallways, and furniture arrangements may all be barriers. Wheelchairs can fit through most front doors, but turning in narrow hallways and small rooms (especially a bathroom) may be impossible. Contractors may be able to widen the doorways and refit a bathroom. Expect scrapes and nicks to appear if a patient has problems handling the wheelchair. Wall corners may be protected with inexpensive, hard plastic molding available from hardware stores. Offset hinges may enable doors to swing clearly, adding an extra inch of space and perhaps preventing the need to rebuild an entire doorway.

Bathrooms are usually the one place in the home that can't accommodate wheelchairs. Often the only bathroom in the house is located on the second floor. The least expensive alternative to remodeling a bathroom is to invest in a commode with armrests. Even for patients who do not use wheelchairs, a commode may be the most practical choice. The downside to this option is that someone has to carry the commode basin to the toilet to empty it.

In the bathroom, a raised toilet seat may help ease transfers. Some DME toilet seats have armrests for safety and to help with transfers. A shower chair may provide a measure of safety for an unsteady person. Tub benches permit bathing while providing leverage when it is time to lift the patient out of the tub. Sturdy bars, installed diagonally rather than vertically or horizontally, should be installed in both showers and tubs. Especially in the bathroom, throw rugs should be removed to prevent tripping and falling.

Other household modifications include intercoms, buzzers, and other signaling devices that not only are useful forms of communication but also provide patients with a sense of security when they are left alone. Floor coverings may need to be reassessed. It's amazing how well patients may be able to walk with a walker on a tile floor in a hospital but at home may bog down in shag carpets as if they were walking in mud.

Occupational therapists can suggest numerous other home modifications based on a patient's needs. Some are simple. Others are quite sophisticated and beyond the price range of many people.

Stroke often causes problems with walking, balance, strength and coordination. The pool can be a perfect setting to make improvements. The water resistance builds strength.
Cheryl, 26
Physical Therapist

Personal Equipment

Patients may be taught *hemidressing,* using the working arm to dress. Obesity, arthritis, poor balance, or weakness may interfere with their ability to reach down and grasp clothes, socks, or shoes. A dressing stick or reacher stick can help patients grab articles of clothing and even maneuver them into place. Sock donners can help with socks. Elastic shoelaces or shoes with hook-and-loop fasteners may eliminate tedious and cumbersome tying. Even something as simple as a long-handled shoehorn can make life easier and promote independence. Use of multiple home-assist devices may be necessary to achieve optimum functioning. Practice using these items is critical but often overlooked. It may initially take patients nearly an hour to dress. They may be very frustrated. The aids may seem cumbersome. But, like any motor skill, speed and accuracy should improve over time.

Arm slings may provide some relief when a stroke patient's arm is immobile and hangs limply to the side. The pull of gravity may stretch tendons, soft tissue, and nerves, resulting in rotator cuff pain. Some patients, however, see such devices as visible signs of disability and are reluctant to use them. The unfortunate result is more pain for these patients. Physicians often find themselves reminding patients that gravity doesn't give up or take time off. Therefore, slings should be worn as directed during walking, transfers, and sometimes in the wheelchair. Creative people may decorate the fabric and perhaps even construct several slings in fabrics that match a patient's clothing.

Like slings, *lapboards* can support the arms. Lapboards are small tables that attach to the wheelchair frame in front of the armrests. Foam wedges placed under the hands may also help reduce swelling in the hands, allowing gravity to drain some of the fluid.

Fluid may build up in paralyzed limbs if they remain immobile. Muscles cannot "pump" blood and other fluids back through the body. At the same time, gravity draws the blood and other fluids downward. Fluid buildup can limit joint motion. Devices such as compression gloves and stockings, which inflate and deflate, help squeeze fluid from the limbs. If there is a lot of fluid (especially in the legs), these devices may be very difficult for the patient's home caregiver to put on and probably impossible for the patient to put on independently. The compressive stockings that patients use in the hospital to prevent blood clots usually can't provide enough compression to drive out much fluid. Sometimes, the easiest way to compress the legs is to use four-inch elastic wraps. However, these wraps gradually lose compression and need to be rewrapped about every four hours.

Transfer boards, which act as a bridge between one surface and another, are helpful for patients who are unable to stand. They are useful for transfers from beds to wheelchairs, wheelchairs to cars, and wheelchairs to toilets. Some patients are able to stand with help but are unable to take many steps or make turns. *Pivot disks,* large plastic disks with ball-bearing bases, may help these patients. Transfer boards and pivot disks are important because they help reduce physical strain on the caregiver and may facilitate mobility without assistance from others.

Inexpensive picture boards or alphabet boards may help bridge some stroke patients' language barriers. Others may be able to learn to use laptop computers and small printers. Newer models can understand the human voice and can print the spoken word. Such aids are referred to as *augmentative communication devices.* Because these electronic devices are expensive and usually not covered by insurance, it is advisable to obtain a speech pathologist's evaluation of a patient's abilities before such a purchase is considered.

Look around for the right rehabilitation hospital. I came to rehab in a wheelchair and later could walk. Four years later, I use the pool and gym to continue making improvements, even though progress is slow. Now that I have adaptive equipment for my car, I hope to drive again.
Donald
Age 74

Plate guards, adapted eating and cooking utensils, hand braces, writing utensils, lever-type door handles and other adaptive items are available and must be tailored to each patient's needs. Spending time with a therapist to find and fit appropriate durable medical equipment can save both money and frustration.

Part IV

Preventing Strokes

11

Reducing Your Risk of Stroke

Every fifty-three seconds, someone in the United States has a stroke. That's about 500,000 new or recurrent strokes each year. Most who suffer strokes are over age sixty-five. Stroke is the third leading cause of death in the United States. Approximately 150,000 to 200,000 individuals die as a direct result of stroke. Stroke is also the most common reason for adult disability. In 1997, more than 3,890,000 people in the United States were living with the effects of stroke. Eighty percent of the population has a family member who will have a stroke or will have a friend living with the effects of stroke. Stroke-related care may cost the country as much as $17 billion each year in direct costs (medical treatment) and another $13 billion in indirect costs (loss of job and income).

Risk Factors

Based on medical statistics and research, we know the risk factors that most frequently cause stroke are hypertension, diabetes, smoking, and some heart problems. Other diseases and lifestyle choices also influence the occurrence of stroke, as shown in the table below. Identifying these conditions and making appropriate lifestyle changes may significantly reduce one's risk of stroke.

Table 3. Risk Factors for Stroke	Risk
Atrial fibrillation plus rheumatic heart disease	18 times
Prior stroke/TIA	10 times
High blood pressure	6 times
Atrial fibrillation	6 times
Congestive heart failure	5 times
Heart attack/angina/sudden death syndrome	3 times
Diabetes mellitus	2-4 times
Heavy alcohol use	2-4 times
Smoking	2-4 times

High Blood Pressure

Uncontrolled *hypertension,* or high blood pressure, is a major cause of stroke. Hypertension is an elevated pressure of blood flow against the walls of the arteries. The most common symptom of high blood pressure is no symptom at all. It's a silent killer. Undiagnosed hypertension can result in strokes, heart attacks, kidney damage, bleeding into the eyes, and even death.

Blood pressure is measured by assessing the force, or pressure, of blood flow inside the arteries during both the contraction and relaxation phases of the heart's pumping cycle. The measurement of blood pressure is stated using two numerals. For example, an individual may have a blood pressure reading of

140/90, which is at the top level of the normal range. The top number, the *systolic value*, is related to heart muscle contraction. The bottom number, the *diastolic value*, relates to the cardiac relaxation cycle. A person is considered to have high blood pressure that should be medically treated and monitored if, after several blood pressure readings, either of these numbers is consistently high.

Reducing salt, or *sodium chloride*, in the diet may help lower blood pressure. Salt increases blood pressure because the body senses the elevated sodium level as abnormal. If excess sodium is present, the body will store water to dilute the sodium. The final effect is similar to adding water to a balloon: the greater the amount of water, the more pressure is on the artery walls. Just like a balloon, excessive blood pressure can burst through a weakness in a vessel wall, causing a hemorrhagic stroke. Most processed foods contain extra salt. Check food labels to determine the amount while you are shopping. You may be surprised at how much salt is in seemingly harmless products.

Sometimes you don't realize that you've had a stroke. My husband developed a leg weakness and just thought it was his arthritis. My mother had mini strokes, and it was difficult to tell when they were occurring.

Brenda
Age 45

Medications may be used to lower blood pressure to normal limits to significantly reduce the risk of stroke. Lowering the diastolic blood pressure by six points may reduce the risk of stroke by 38 to 42 percent. Unfortunately, some people may experience unpleasant side effects from certain medications. If this happens, doctors may prescribe alternatives. It is critical that a person who is taking blood pressure medication not change the dose nor discontinue taking it without first talking with a physician. This is especially true for the elderly. Even if they have never shown any signs of high blood pressure, people over the age of fifty have an increased risk of developing high blood pressure. Why? Their blood vessels tend to lose elasticity with age. Blood pressure must be carefully monitored, even while taking medication, to prevent it from dropping too low and depriving the brain of blood or rising so high that blood vessels burst. Biofeedback, visual imagery, and relaxation therapy may also help people lower their blood pressure.

Atherosclerosis

Atherosclerosis—hardening of the arteries—results from a diet high in fat, usually from animal sources like beef and pork. This fat, *atherosclerotic plaque*, may attach itself to arteries as it travels through the body. Eventually, blood vessels may become blocked. The tissue upstream may not receive the nourishment it needs to live. Atherosclerotic plaque may fragment, travel through the body, lodge in the brain, and cause a stroke. This is especially true of plaque originating in the neck arteries or the ascending aorta, the large artery that arises from the heart and feeds the neck arteries.

To prevent strokes in patients suspected of having atherosclerotic blockage, a *Doppler test* can be performed on the carotid arteries in the neck. During this procedure, sound waves are bounced off the artery walls to check for abnormal or absent blood flow. If a blockage is detected, and the person is medically stable enough for an operation, a vascular surgeon may order an *arteriogram.* A special fluid that shows up on X-rays is injected into the arteries. This test helps further define areas of narrowed or clogged vessels. If the patient's arteries have 60 to 70 percent or more blockage, a *carotid endarterectomy* operation may be performed to open the artery and remove the cholesterol. This is a major surgical procedure with risks that include stroke if the plaque breaks loose. Generally, men seem to fare better with this procedure than women.

Periodic blood cholesterol tests can help monitor the risk of atherosclerosis. In general, blood cholesterol levels should be below 200 milligrams per deciliter. Reducing fat in the diet is one of the best ways to reduce cholesterol levels. However, in certain cases, medications may be prescribed to lower the blood fats and cholesterol. These drugs are especially useful for people diagnosed with a hereditary form of atherosclerosis. However, some individuals may have fat levels in the blood that are hard to control even with medication and a modified diet.

Atrial Fibrillation

As noted in an earlier chapter, *atrial fibrillation*, is a disease of the *atrium*, the upper left heart chamber. It causes an irregular heart rate and rhythm. In a normal heart, the atrium contracts and pumps blood into the chamber beneath it, the *ventricle*. The ventricle then contracts and forces blood into general circulation. If the atrium is diseased, it may begin to quiver rather than pump. Blood that is not squeezed into the ventricle may sludge and form clots. If the clots break loose, they may circulate and lodge in the brain, causing a stroke. There is also a higher risk that clots may continue to be thrown from the heart, producing more strokes. Strokes resulting from atrial fibrillation tend to be severe, doubling the risk of death within the first month. When a clot breaks loosse from the heart, it can fragment and damage multiple areas in the brain. Atrial fibrillation also tends to increase after age fifty. Atrial fibrillation may be suspected if a *computerized axial tomography (CAT)* or *magnetic resonance imaging (MRI) scan* shows multiple areas of the brain affected by the stroke.

Still, atrial fibrillation may be difficult to detect because the heart may alternate between fibrillation and normal rhythms. So a patient may be asked to wear a small, portable heart monitor for an entire day to check for atrial fibrillation or other abnormal heart rhythms. In some people atrial fibrillation may be chronic (lasting more than six months) and may not respond to medical therapy. Aspirin and warfarin, anticoagulant medications, may prevent clotting. Yet both have the potential to cause other bleeding problems. Other medications are available to regulate heart rhythms. Cardiologists may elect to try a *cardioversion*, which uses an electrical charge to convert the rhythm of the heart back to normal.

> *If we had known the signs of stroke, it would have helped us realize sooner that my husband was having a stroke. Immediate medical attention can make such a difference.*
> *Ellen*
> *Age 49*

Coagulation Disorders

Problems with *coagulation,* or blood clotting, inside arteries serving the brain or the heart may cause a stroke. The body is always working to break up any clots that may form. However, certain chemistries in the body may make one prone to clots. These clots may, in turn, bring on a stroke. Coagulation disorders are difficult to isolate. Even thorough testing may miss the subtle changes in blood chemistry that may indicate a tendency toward clotting.

Other strokes may be caused by *vasculitis,* a condition in which blood vessels within the brain become so inflamed and swollen that blood flow is restricted. Both coagulation disorders and vasculitis respond to the drug warfarin, which helps prevent new clots.

Smoking

Smoking is a major risk factor for strokes. The substances in tobacco affect not only the lungs but also blood circulation. The more a person smokes, the greater the risk of permanent damage to the body. Smoking has been shown to lead to high blood pressure, strokes, heart attacks, emphysema, and lung cancer. It may contribute to atherosclerosis, diminishing blood flow to the brain. In a study of more than 7,000 men over thirteen years of age smokers had four times as many strokes as nonsmokers. People who smoke two or more packs of cigarettes per day have twice the risk of stroke as those who smoke less than half a pack per day.

My son wouldn't take care of his high blood pressure and didn't control his weight. If he had, I think his stroke could have been prevented.

Joyce
Age 56

Smoking is a complex behavior encompassing both nicotine addiction and habitual behavioral patterns. Physicians have an array of tools—from prescription medications to behavior modification methods—to help people who truly want to quit. Some smoking cessation medications like nicotine gum and nicotine patches no longer require a prescription. For the best chance of success, these aids may need to be combined with a supportive formal smoking cessation program. Most communities offer such programs. It usually takes several serious attempts before someone finally quits smoking. It is encouraging that, after five years, people who have quit smoking have the same risk of stroke as nonsmokers.

Obesity

Obesity doesn't necessarily lead directly to a stroke. But the presence of a lot of fat tissue means the body has to make more blood vessels to nourish the tissue. And the heart has to work harder to pump blood. This extra work may contribute to high blood pressure and congestive heart failure, both risk factors for stroke.

Oral Contraceptives

Research suggests that birth-control pills may cause stroke, especially in women over thirty-five who smoke. It is believed that the estrogen in birth-control pills may cause clots that lead to stroke. Accordingly, in recent years, the estrogen content in birth-control pills has been lowered. Medication with less estrogen works just as effectively as a contraceptive and probably lowers the risk of stroke. It does not, however, completely eliminate the risk.

Alcohol Consumption

Studies indicate that light to heavy use of alcohol may increase by two to three times the chance of a bleeding stroke. Heavy drinkers have up to four times the risk of experiencing a subarachnoid hemorrhagic stroke.

Other Risk Factors

People who have *obstructive sleep apnea*, a condition that causes breathing to temporarily stop during sleep, may experience drops in blood oxygen levels that may initiate strokes.

After a stroke, the risk of death increases for diabetics, the elderly, those with severe neurological deficits from previous strokes, and individuals who have had heart attacks or have abnormal heart rhythms. Small blood clots, or *microemboli*, may cause strokes. These small clots may be caused by artificial heart valves, atrial fibrillation, heart attacks, and narrowing of the carotid arteries.

Is heredity a factor in risk of strokes? It is hard to scientifically prove specific hereditary risk factors for strokes since they may be caused by so many different factors.

I became a statistic. I had a stroke. I am angry with myself for thirty-five years of destructive cigarette smoking. After a stroke, your priorities in life change. You develop a greater sense of love for yourself and others.

Kathy
Age 49

Risk of Recurrent Strokes

There is a 10 to 18 percent risk of having a second stroke in the first year immediately following a stroke. The risk continues to grow about 10 percent each following year. Most people may expect to live eight years after a first stroke.

One of the major causes of recurrent stroke is a lack of change in lifestyle. Some people may not monitor their blood pressure or take care of their diabetes or may continue to smoke. Failure to take prescribed stroke medication is another significant cause of recurrence. Some patients stop medications because they don't like the expense. Others may stop because of side effects.

Doctors and family members should encourage stroke patients to take all prescribed medications.

The Importance of Exercise

When my wife's stroke hit, it was scary. She just sat there, staring at a blank television screen. She jumbled all her words...like she was saying them backwards. She had problems from the stroke for about six months.

Tom
Age 39

Regular and appropriate exercise not only increases circulation and lung capacity but also fights cholesterol buildup. Reducing the risk of stroke also seems to depend on the amount of exercise. Exercise needs to be regular and should reach an individual's *target heart rate* for maximum benefit. To calculate target heart rate, subtract your age from 220, then multiply that value by 60 to 70 percent. Ideally, you should maintain your target heart rate for thirty minutes, three times per week. It is wise to check with a physician before starting an aerobic exercise program if you have a medical condition like congestive heart failure, heart attack, heart beat irregularities, and/or asthma. A doctor may recommend that exercise be undertaken with appropriate supervision, such as that offered at a cardiac rehabilitation center.

Facts About Strokes

The U.S. Center for Disease Control, National Institute of Health, and the American Heart Association collect statistics from around the country to help the medical and scientific community determine who is most at risk of stroke. Some of their findings are listed here.

- Stroke is the leading cause of serious, long-term disability in the United States.
- Stroke accounts for more than half of all patients hospitalized for acute neurological disease.
- Thirty-one percent of stroke survivors needed help caring for themselves, 20 percent needed help walking, and 71 percent had an impaired vocational capacity when examined an average of 7 years later. Sixteen percent were institutionalized.
- The vast majority of strokes occur after age sixty-five. Thus, age is the biggest factor in developing a stroke.
- About 28 percent of strokes occur in persons under age 65.

Facts About Strokes (con't)

- For people over age 55, the incidence of stroke more than doubles in each successive decade.
- The incidence of stroke is about 19 percent higher for males than for females.
- African-Americans' chances of stroke are about double those of whites.
- People in the southeastern United States have a higher incidence of stroke than those in the rest of the country.
- Risks for stroke are higher for people whose parents had strokes.
- Females comprise nearly 61 percent of stroke fatalities. More than 91,000 women die each year of stroke, while lung cancer claims 57,600.
- For white males, the death rate from stroke is about 27 percent.
- For black males, the death rate from stroke is about 52 percent, 94 percent greater than for whites.
- White females have a 23 percent risk of death from stroke.
- Black females have a 40 percent risk of death from stroke, 76 percent higher than white females.

Resources

Hospitals, rehab centers, doctors, therapists, and other professionals can provide resource materials and references to information about stroke. Local and state health departments usually have materials that can be helpful. The internet has abundant information about stroke. Also, the following organizations provide public information about stroke and recovery.

National Stroke Association
    8480 E. Orchard Rd., Suite 1000
    Englewood, CO 80111-5015
    (303) 649-9299
    1-800-STROKES (787-6537)
    fax (303) 649-1328
    www.stroke.org
    National Stroke Association (NSA) is a national voluntary
    health care organization focusing on stroke prevention,
    treatment, rehabilitation, research and support for stroke
    survivors and their families. NSA offers information and
    materials on public education, professional education,
    treatment, research and stroke survivor/caregiver support and

resources, books, newsletters, brochures, videos, posters, slides, and more.

Stroke Connection/American Heart Association National Center
7272 Greenville Ave.
Dallas, TX 75231-4596
1-800-553-6321
www.amhrt.org

American Health Assistance Foundation
15825 Shady Grove Road, Suite 140
Rockville, MD 20850
Phone: 1-800-437-2423
Phone: (301) 948-3244
Fax (301) 258-9454
http://www.ahaf.org/

American Institute of Stress
124 Park Ave.
Yonkers, NY 10703
Phone (914) 963-1200
Fax (914) 965-6267
www.stress.org
e-mail: stress124@earthlink.net

National Heart, Lung, and Blood Institute
National Institutes of Health
http://www.nhlbi.nih.gov/nhlbi/nhlbi.htm
National Institute of Neurological Disorders and Stroke
National Institutes of Health
Bethesda, MD 20892
http://www.ninds.nih.gov/

National Institute of Neurological Disorders and Stroke
Office of Scientific and Health Reports
P.O. Box 5801
Bethesda, MD 20824
Phone: (301) 496-5751
Phone: 1-800-352-9424
http://www.ninds.nih.gov/healinfo/disorder/stroke/agencies.ht

NARIC National Rehabilitation Information Center
National Institute on Disability and Rehabilitation Research
8455 Colesville Road, Suite 935
Silver Spring, MD 20910-3319
800-346-2742 (V)
(301) 588-9284 (V)
(301) 495-5626 (TT)
(301) 587-1967 (fax)
http://www.naric.com/naric

Office on Smoking and Health (OSH)
National Center for Chronic Disease Prevention and Health
Promotion (NCCDPHP)
Centers for Disease Control and Prevention (CDC)
4770 Buford Highway, NE
Mail Stop K-50
Atlanta, Georgia 30341-3724
Phone: (770) 488-5705
1-800-CDC-1311 (Voice/Fax Information)
Internet: http://www.cdc.gov/tobacco
E-mail: ccdinfo@cdc.gov

American Lung Association
1740 Broadway
New York, New York 10019-4374
1-800-LUNG-USA

National Rehabilitation Information Center (NARIC)
  http://www.naric.com/naric/search.

U.S. Department of Health and Human Services
  Public Health Service Agency for Health Care Policy and
    Research
  Executive Office Center, Suite 501
  2101 East Jefferson Street
  Rockville, MD 20852
  http://www.healthtouch.com

Agency for Health Care Policy and Research (AHCPR)
  http://www.medlib.com/ahcpr
  AHCPR Publications Clearinghouse
  P.O. Box 8547
  Silver Spring, MD 20907
  1-800-358-9295.

American Heart Association
  7272 Greenville Avenue
  Dallas, TX 75231
  (214) 373-6300
  (800) 242-8721

Agency for Health Care Policy and Research
  P.O. Box 8547
  Silver Spring, MD 20907
  (800) 358-9295

Institute for Health and Disability
  University of Minnesota, Box 721
  420 Delaware Street, SE
  Minneapolis, MN 55455-0392
  (612) 626-2825

National Institute on Deafness and Other Communication Disorders
  Building 31, Room 3C35

Bethesda, MD 20892-2320
(301) 496-7243
Provides education, research, information, and referrals.
sponsors a speakers bureau, workshops, and conferences.
Publishes pamphlets, brochures, booklets, a newsletter, and a
professional journal. Sponsors nationwide chapters and
support groups.

The Department of Health and Human Services
Hubert H. Humphrey Building
200 Independence Avenue SW
Washington, D.C., 20201.
www.os.dhhs.gov
The Department of Health and Human Services is the United
States government's principal agency for protecting the health
of all Americans and providing essential human services,
especially for those who are least able to help themselves. The
department includes more than 300 programs, covering a wide
spectrum of activities. Services include: Medical and social
science research, Medicare (health insurance for elderly and
disabled Americans) and Medicaid (health insurance for
low-income citizens), financial assistance for low-income
families (AFDC), services for older Americans, including
home-delivered meals.

Universities with stroke research centers:
Washington University School of Medicine, St. Louis, Missouri
Mayo Foundation, Rochester, Minnesota
The Johns Hopkins University, Baltimore, Maryland
University of Maryland School of Medicine, Baltimore, Maryland
Cornell University Medical Center, New York, New York
University of Pennsylvania, Philadelphia, Pennsylvania
Massachusetts General Hospital, Boston, Massachusetts
Oregon Health Sciences University, Portland, Oregon

University of Texas Medical School, Houston, Texas
University of Iowa College of Medicine, Iowa City, Iowa
University of Miami School of Medicine, Miami, Florida
University of California, Los Angeles, California
University of California, San Francisco, California
Bowman Gray School of Medicine at Wake Forest University,
    Winston-Salem, North Carolina
Henry Ford Hospital, Detroit, Michigan

Glossary

A

Activities of Daily Living (ADLs): Daily functions of dressing, eating, walking, hygiene, going to the toilet, and communication

Acute medical care: The initial phases of care after a stroke in which the patient is stabilized and diagnostic studies are begun

Aftercare: The processes of arranging discharge and outpatient needs

Agnosia: Inability to recognize things

Ambulation: Walking or gait

Amnesia: Inability to remember certain things

Anemia: Less than normal amount of circulating red blood cells

Aneurysm: Small, bubble-like protrusion from the side of a blood vessel; this weakness can rupture and cause a stroke

Angina: Chest pain from lack of oxygen reaching the heart; this can be the warning sign of a heart attack

Angiography: An X-ray in which contrast dye is injected into the artery to "light up" arteries to evaluate sites of bleeding, blocked or spasming vessels

Ankle-Foot Orthosis (AFO): Plastic or metal short-leg brace

Anomia: Inability to name objects, yet having ability to use and describe them

Anosognosia: Brain damage that results in denying or neglecting deficits

Anoxic encephalopathy: Brain damage from a type of stroke due to insufficient blood pressure

Anterior cerebral artery: An artery running up the front of the cerebrum

Anticoagulants: Oral and intravenous medications which block the formation of blood clots

Anticoagulation: The process of preventing clot formation within blood vessels

Anticonvulsant: Medication used to treat and prevent seizures

Antidepressant: Medication used to treat depression

Aphasia: A complex disturbance in expression and/or understanding of speech and language

Apraxia: Inability to perform a *directed* action, yet having physical ability to do the action

Arteriogram: Test in which contrast dye is injected into arteries to look for abnormalities such as narrowing

Arteriovenous malformation: Abnormal collection of blood vessels where arteries feed directly into veins without the usual capillaries in between; this creates an abnormal pressure situation that can allow bleeding into the brain

Arthritis: Painful inflammation of joints

Aspiration: When food or fluid is inhaled into the lungs instead of traveling down the normal swallowing tube

Aspirin: A nonsteroid anti-inflammatory medication used as an anticoagulant by inhibiting platelet clotting

Ataxia: Loss of coordination

Glossary

Atelectasis: Small airway collapse in the lungs

Atherosclerosis: Deposition of fat into the walls of arteries which eventually reduces the diameter of the vessel and blocks blood flow

Atria: The two upper chambers of the heart

Atrial fibrillation: An abnormal heart rhythm; this can allow blood to sludge within the heart and can allow formation of a clot

Augmentative communication: Use of devices, like a computer, to assist patients in communication

B

Behavior: A person's actions and reactions

Bladder: Bag-like storage organ for urine which contracts to empty

Bolus: Food or fluid formed into a ball by the mouth so it can be swallowed

Bowel: Long tubular abdominal organ which stores and empties feces

Brainstem: A lower area of the brain which is part of the involuntary nervous system and controls some functions necessary for life

Broca's aphasia: The inability to express language

C

Cardiologist: Doctor specializing in diseases/disorders of the heart and circulatory system

Cardiopulmonary resuscitation: Technique of artificial breathing and chest compressions used for people whose heart and lung function has stopped

Cardioversion: The process of applying an electrical charge to the chest wall to convert a patient's abnormal heart rhythm into a normal rhythm

Carotid arteries: Paired arteries moving blood from the heart through the neck and into the head; it is often blocked by atherosclerotic plaque

Carotid endarterectomy: An operation to remove atherosclerotic plaque from the carotid artery to allow a clear channel for blood flow

Case manager: Specialist in assisting with admissions/discharges and social aspects of rehabilitation care

CAT Scan (Computerized Axial Tomography): Sophisticated radiologic test to show the anatomy of internal body parts

Catheter: A plastic tube inserted into the bladder to passively drain urine

Central intravenous line: A plastic tube inserted into a large vein in the neck to allow delivery of nutrition, medications and fluid

Cerebellum: The back part of the brain which controls coordination

Cerebrospinal fluid: Nutritional fluid which circulates within and around the brain and spinal cord

Cerebrovascular accident (CVA): Stroke

Cerebrum: The upper part of the brain which helps control thinking and voluntary action

Cholesterol: Fatty substance that can collect in the walls of arteries and block the flow of blood

Circle of Willis: A protective ring of blood vessels at the base of the brain

Clonus: A rapid, alternating motion of the ankle from spasticity

Coagulation: The process of forming a clot within a blood vessel

Cognition: The processes involved with thinking

Collateral flow: Where blood flow from other vessels substitutes for blood that is blocked in another vessel

Coma: Unconscious state from which a person cannot be aroused

Comorbidity: Other diseases a patient may have, some of which may impact on the effects of a stroke

Constipation: Poor ability to evacuate the bowel

Glossary

Contact guard assist level: Caregiver has hands-on touch with the patient while a task is performed

Contraceptives (oral): Birth control pills

Contractures: Soft tissue shortening which restricts joint motion

Convulsions: See epilepsy

Cortex or cortical area: The outer most layer of the cerebrum

Cortical blindness: Damage to the back part of the brain (occipital lobes) that causes a person to not recognize their blindness

Cranial nerves: Twelve pairs of nerves that function in the head and neck for smell, taste, swallow, tongue/face/eye motion and vision/hearing

Cryptogenic stroke: Stroke due to an undetermined cause

D

Decubitus ulcers: Skin breakdown from excessive pressure or shear forces

Deep vein thrombosis: Blood clots in the leg which can break free and travel to the lungs causing a pulmonary embolus

Deficits: Problems with functioning

Dementia: Deterioration of mental processes

Dependent level of assist: Caretakers are doing all tasks for a patient

Depression: Feelings of helplessness, hopelessness, despair and possibly thoughts of suicide

Diabetes mellitus: A complex metabolic disturbance, especially of blood sugars

Diarrhea: Thin, loose stool

Diastolic value: The bottom number of the blood pressure reading

Diplopia: Double-vision caused by damage to certain cranial nerves so the eyes do not work together

Disability: How an impairment affects ability to perform certain usual life functions

Diuretic: Also called a "water pill" because it causes loss of water from the body

Dizziness: Light-headed sensation

Dopplers: A noninvasive test to determine blood flow in a vessel

Durable medical equipment (DME): Equipment used for long-term needs, such as a wheelchair or walker

Dysarthria: Slurred speech because of weak or absent function of muscles

Dysfunction: Poor function

Dysphagia: Difficulty with swallowing

E

Echocardiogram: A test using sound waves to look for heart abnormalities

Edema: Swelling

Electroconvulsive therapy (ECT): A treatment for depression in which an electrical impulse is applied to the brain

Electroencephalogram (EEG): A test of brain waves to check for seizures, brain damage and brain death

Elevated walker: A type of walker with a raised pad/hand grips to allow the patient to bear some weight through the pad

Embolism: Blood clot that has broken free and traveled downstream in a blood vessel until it lodges and clogs a vessel

Emotional lability: Inability to control the emotions

Enema: Putting fluid into the rectum to produce a bowel movement

Engrams: A patterned nerve-muscle loop developed over multiple repetitions which builds up coordination

Epiglottis: A flap of tissue which folds down to protect the open airway during swallowing

Epilepsy: A disorder in which the brain produces spontaneous discharges which usually alter consciousness and cause convulsions

Equilibrium: Sense of balance

Esophagus: Swallowing tube running from the throat to the stomach

F

Family practitioner: Doctor specializing in diseases/disorders of all ages

Figure-ground perception: Ability to distinguish between objects that are near versus far or distinct versus less formed

Foot drop: The foot drops down as the result of weak muscles on the front part of the lower leg

Frontal lobes: Paired lobes in the front part of the cerebrum

Functional range of motions: Joint mobility sufficient to do normal tasks

Functional recovery: The return of abilities like eating, walking and dressing

G

Gait: Walking or ambulation

Gait belt: A strong belt placed around a patient's waist to assist with transfers and walking

Gastrocolic reflex: A reflex of the bowels which pushes stool along the colon after intake of new food

Gastrostomy tube (G-tube or PEG tube): A flexible tube surgically placed through the stomach wall to safely provide liquid food and water

Gaze preference: Tendency to look in one direction due to a visual field cut

Global aphasia: The most severe form of aphasia in which the ability to speak and understand language is nearly or completely disrupted

Grand mal seizure: See tonic-clonic seizure

H

Heart attack (myocardial infarction): Death of heart muscle when it is deprived of oxygen

Hemianopsia: Loss of one-half of a visual field

Hemicane: A large based, four-legged device used to assist with walking the patient who has poor balance

Hemidressing techniques: Methods used to teach a patient with hemiplegia how to dress

Hemiplegia: Weakness or paralysis of the same-side arm and leg

Hemisphere: Half of the cerebrum or half of the cerebellum

Hemorrhage: Bleeding outside of the blood vessels

Hemorrhoids: Enlarged blood vessels in the anus/rectal region which can bleed and be painful

Heparin: A type of anticoagulant given by intravenous or intramuscular injection

Herniation: Protrusion of a body part out of its normal cavity

Hydrocephalus: Accumulation of extra fluid within the cavities of the brain

Hypercoagulable state: Condition where the body forms an excessive amount of blood clots, which can predispose to strokes

Hypertension: High blood pressure

Hypotension: Low blood pressure

I

Immobilization syndrome: The deconditioning effects of prolonged bed rest or illness that decrease a person's strength and endurance

Impotence: Inability of a man to produce an erection

Incontinence: Inability to control bowel or bladder function, resulting in spilling fecal matter or urine

Independent level: The patient is able to do all of a task alone

Indwelling catheter: A plastic tube which stays in the bladder to drain it

Infarction: Tissue death due to extreme lack of oxygen

Inferior vena cava filter: A filter placed in the large vein leading to the heart for the purpose of stopping dangerous blood clots in the legs from reaching the heart and lungs

Inhibition: A signal to a muscle preventing its movement; a signal restricting a behavior

Intellect: The ability to learn, understand and act in a purposeful manner

Intermittent catheterization: Bladder program of inserting a tube into the bladder at intervals, then removing it

Internist or internal medicine physician: Doctor specializing in diseases/disorders of adults

Intracerebral hemorrhage: Bleeding into the substance of the brain

Intravenous line (IV): A plastic tube inserted into the veins to provide fluid and to give a route to deliver medication

Intraventricular hemorrhage: Bleeding into the deep cavities of the brain

Ischemia: Relative lack of oxygen in tissues

J

Jejunostomy tube (J-tube): An artificial feeding tube surgically placed into the second part of the small intestine

Joint contractures: See contractures

K

Knee-Ankle-Foot Orthosis (KAFO): Plastic or metal long-leg brace

L

Lacunar stroke: Tissue death due to small vessel disease in the deep parts of the brain

Lapboard: Flat board which sits across the wheelchair armrests to allow the patient to use arms more easily

Level of assistance: The amount of help that is required for a task

Locked-in syndrome: Type of stroke due to damage at the base of the pons in the brainstem; patient cannot move or communicate except for eye blinks

M

Magnetic Resonance Image: Complicated radiologic test to detect abnormalities of internal organs

Mass effect: Pressure effect from bleeding or swelling reaction of damaged brain tissue that forces parts of the brain to move away from the pressure

Maximum assist level: Caregivers are helping with 75 percent of a task

Melodic intonation therapy: A speech therapy technique of having the patient sing to stimulate better ability to speak

Microemboli: Very small blood clots which can cause strokes

Middle cerebral artery: An artery serving the middle portion of the brain

Minimal assist level: Caregivers are helping with 25 percent of a task

Mitral valve prolapse: Heart condition in which the mitral valves collapse inward instead of preventing the back flow of blood; thought to be a possible source of emboli

Moderate assist level: Caregivers are helping with 50 percent of a task

Modified barium swallow: See videofluoroscopy

Morbidity: Diseased or damaged state

Mortality: Death

Muscle rotation flap: A plastic surgery procedure—muscle, skin and its blood supply are rotated to cover a large decubitus ulcer area

Musculoskeletal: Pertaining to the muscles, ligaments, tendons and bones

Myocardial infarction: See heart attack

N

Nasogastric (NG) tube: A flexible plastic tube inserted into the nose and down into the stomach, used for those with swallowing disorders

Neglect: Tendency to ignore or to be unaware of part of the environment

Neurogenic bladder: Damage to the brain resulting in bladder control problems

Neurologic recovery: Healing and return of function of the nervous system

Neuron: A nerve cell

Nursing home care: A level of medical care involving less intense therapy

O

Occipital lobes: Paired lobes in the back part of the cerebrum

Occupational therapy (OT): Specialty designed to restore arm function, cognition, activities of daily living and help with adaptive equipment

Ophthalmologist: Doctor specializing in diseases/disorders of vision

Oral contraceptives: Birth control pills

Orthosis: A brace for the arm, leg, neck or spine

Orthotist: Specialist in making and fitting braces

P

Parietal lobes: Paired lobes in the upper sides of the cerebrum

PEG (percutaneous endoscopic gastrostomy) tube: A gastrostomy tube

Penetration: Food/fluid traveling down to the level of the vocal cords

Perception: The ability to know things by interacting with the environment

Peripheral vascular disease: The process of atherosclerosis excluding the heart arteries

Perseveration: Repetitive vocalization of same words or thoughts

Physiatrist: Doctor specializing in physical medicine and rehabilitation

Physical Therapy (PT): Specialty designed to help regain strength, coordination, balance, walking, endurance

Plastic surgeon: Surgical specialist dealing with skin and underlying structures

Plasticity: The potential of a healthy part of the brain taking over the functions of the damaged portion

Platelet-derived growth factor: Part of a patient's own blood which is harvested and grown to then be placed over a decubitus ulcer to speed its healing

Platelets: Irregularly shaped granules that circulate in the blood and are part of the formation of blood clots

Pneumonia: Infection of the lung

Pons: Part of the brain stem

Posterior cerebral artery: An artery serving the back parts of the cerebrum

Proprioception: Joint position sense

Prosthetist: Specialist in making and fitting artificial limbs

Glossary

Psychiatrist: Doctor specializing in mental health diseases/disorders

Pulmonary embolism: Blood clot from the leg that has broken loose and travels to the lung

Pulmonologist: Doctor specializing in diseases/disorders of the lungs

Pusher syndrome: Tendency to push with the strong side which can lead to balance problems

Q

Quadrantanopsia: Loss of one-quarter of a visual field

R

Range of motion: Total motion produced at a joint; the process of doing joint motion to prevent joint contractures

Reflex sympathetic dystrophy: Damage to nerves where the sympathetic nerves contribute to a syndrome of pain, swelling and loss of limb function

Rehabilitation: The therapeutic process, trying to make functional gains and prevent the formation of new functional deficits

Respite care: Temporary patient care by another caregiver, while primary caregivers are allowed a rest period

Rheumatic heart disease: Heart valve damage from earlier bacterial infection of the valves which results in emboli formation

S

Seizures: See epilepsy

Shoulder subluxation: The partial separation of the bones of the shoulder joint because of the unopposed pull of gravity

Silent aspiration: When food/fluid enters the lungs without signs of coughing or choking

Skilled care: A level of medical care where the patient may be only able to handle one therapy per day

Sleep apnea: A condition in which breathing stops during sleep and then starts again

Social worker: See case manager

Sodium chloride: Salt

Spasticity: Increased tone of a muscle due to a lack of inhibitory brain control

Speech Pathology: Specialty designed to restore language, and help with cognitive and swallowing problems

Split thickness skin graft: A plastic surgery procedure, transplanting healthy skin to cover a decubitus ulcer

Sprouting: New connections formed between living nerve cells that survive after a stroke

Standby assist level: Caregiver is next to the patient during a task but is not touching the patient unless immediate help is needed

Status epilepticus: A medical emergency in which one seizure is followed by a cycle of seizures

Stroke: An abnormal neurological condition in which blood flow to part of the brain is interrupted, causing nerve damage

Subacute rehabilitation: A less intense rehabilitation program for those who have partially achieved their goals or for those who need to build up strength/endurance enough to participate in a more intense program

Subarachnoid hemorrhage: Bleeding in the subarachnoid brain space when an aneurysm ruptures

Subcortical brain: The cerebral hemisphere regions of the brain below the cortex

Subluxation: Partial loss of contact of the two surfaces contacting within a joint

Suppository: Medication inserted in the rectum

Suprapubic catheter: Surgically created tube placed above the pubic bone to act as a long-term method to drain urine

Sympathetic nervous system: Part of the involuntary nervous system

Glossary

Synaptophysin: A chemical in the brain that helps in strengthening connections between nerve cells

Systolic value: The upper number of a blood pressure reading

T

Temporal lobes: Paired lobes in the lower sides of the cerebrum

Thalamic pain syndrome: Sensation of burning pain in a body part, as a result of damage to the thalamus

Thalamus: A deep region of the subcortical cerebrum which acts as a sensory relay center

Therapeutic Recreation (TR): A specialty designed to assist in return of socialization, thinking, coordination, strength and leisure activities

Thermal stimulation: Speech therapy technique in which a cold stimulus is placed in the lateral/back region of the throat to improve swallowing

Thrombosis: Process of clotting

Thrombus: Clot

Ticlopidine: Medication used to prevent clots that could cause strokes

Todd's paralysis: A paralysis that can last up to twenty-four hours after some seizures

Tone: The resistance of a muscle to passive motion

Tonic-clonic seizure: A dramatic form of epilepsy in which a patient becomes unconscious, shakes uncontrollably, and may be incontinent

Trachea: Windpipe

Tracheostomy: Surgical opening made in the windpipe to place a tube

Transesophageal echocardiography: Test in which a probe is inserted into the swallowing tube to allow ultrasound echo signals to check for clots in the heart

Transfer: The process of moving from one surface to another

Transient Ischemic Attack (TIA): Neurologic deficits that last less than twenty-four hours

Triglycerides: One of the components of fat that circulates in the blood

U

Unmasking: See plasticity

Urethra: Tube leading from the bladder for urination

Urinary tract infection: Infection from bacteria in the bladder or kidney

Urodynamics: Test done by placing a flexible tube in the bladder and inflating it with water or air to determine bladder function

Urologist: Doctor specializing in urinary and male reproductive systems

Urosepsis: Severe form of urinary tract infection

V

Vasculitis: Inflammation of a blood vessel which may cause it to block blood flow

Vasospasm: Constriction of a blood vessel

Ventilation-perfusion scan: A test to detect pulmonary embolus

Ventricles: The four cavities deep within the brain; also, the two lower chambers in the heart

Vertebrobasilar system: Blood flow from the vertebral and basilar arteries which come up the back of the brain and flow into the Circle of Willis

Vertigo: Sensation of spinning around

Vestibular system: Part of nervous system which monitors equilibrium

Videofluoroscopy: Test in which patient takes in food/fluid while an X-ray video camera monitors the travel of the bolus to check for aspiration

Visual field loss: Blind spot

Void: To urinate

W

Warfarin: Medication used as an anticoagulant

Wernicke's aphasia: The inability to understand language

Index

Index

burning sensation 15
bursitis 64

C

canes 83
cardiologists 87, 110
cardiopulmonary
    resuscitation(CPR) 7
cardiversion 110
carotid
    arteries 11, 113
    endarterectomy 109
case managers 84-85, 88
catheter 53
    indwelling 53
    SP 53
    suprapubic 53
central IV line 48
cerebellum 10, 11, 39
cerebral cortex 19
cerebrum 9
cheeks 32, 42
chest pain 60
chin-tilt maneuver 46
choking 42, 49
cholesterol 5, 109
circulatory problems 59-61
clots 4, 5, 6, 8, 20, 59, 61, 75, 101,
    109, 110, 111, 113
    abnormal heart rhythms 6
    artificial heart 6
    heart attack 6
    heart bypass 6
    infections 6
    leg 60
    mitral valve prolapse 6
    rheumatic heart disease 6
clotting abnormalities 7-8

coagulation disorders 110-111
cognition 19, 22
    elements of 19
commands, following 32
commode 99
communication 30, 32, 51
    foundations 33
    intimate 58
    pictorial 31
    problems 14
    skills 27
comorbidity 72
compensatory techniques 20
comprehension 30
auditory 32
compression
    gloves 39, 101
    stockings 66
    wraps 66
computerized axial
    tomography(CAT) 110
concentration 22
concrete thinking 9
confusion 14
congestive heart failure 75, 106
constipation 54, 56
contact guard assist level 81
contractures 66
control, emotion 23
convulsions 62
coordination 10, 11, 15, 37, 39
    center 39
    lack of 15, 39
cortical
    area 9, 63
    blindness 20, 21
cough

tightening 37-38
tone 38
weakness 36
musculoskeletal pain 64

N

nasogastric tubes 47
National Heart, Lung, and Blood
    Institute 118
National Institute of Neurological
    Disorders and Stroke 118
National Rehabilitation Information
    Center(NARIC) 119, 120
National Stroke Association 117
neglect 36
nerves 11
neurologic bladder 53
neurological recovery 72-73
neurologist 62
neuropsychologists 84
NG tube 47, 49, 48, 56,
nicotine addiction 111
nondominant hands 34, 47
NPO (nothing by mouth) 47
numbness 21, 77
    leg 68
    limbs 21
nursing home care 80
nutrition 48

O

obesity 100, 112
obstructive sleep apnea 113
occipital lobe 9, 10, 20
occupational
    therapists 39, 46, 82, 83, 89, 90, 93,
    96, 97, 100
    therapy 80

Office on Smoking and Health 119
opposite side sensation loss 14
opthalmologists 87
oral contraceptives 112
oral stage 43
organization skills 32
orientation 22
    spatial 19
orthotists 82, 86, 94

P

pain 63-65
    loss of sensation 63
    musculoskeletal 64
    rotator cuff 101
panic 28
paralysis 12, 14, 32, 35, 71
    Todd's 62
parietal lobe 9, 21
parallel bars 95
passive range of motion 39
pathways, engram 40
PEG tube 48-49
penetration 42
perception 19-22
personal equipment 100-102
personality change 23, 24
pharyngeal stage 43, 46
physiatrist 82
physical
    therapists(PTs) 82, 89, 90, 93
    therapy 80
pictorial communication boards 31
picture boards 102
pivot disks 102
plaque 108
plastic surgeons 87
plasticity 33, 77

brain 40, 45
ventilation-perfusion 60
scar tissue 73
seizures 15, 61-63
grand mal 62
self
care skills 30
esteem 26
image 22, 57
pity 57
sensation 9
loss, opposite side 14
burning 15
facial 57
loss of 12
touch 15, 22
pain 63
sensory loss 15
sex organs 57
sexual problems 50, 57-58
sexuality 22
urinary devices 58
shoulder subluxation 64
silent aspiration 43, 44, 45
single-point cane 95
skilled care 79, 80
skin
elasticity 66
graft 67
problems 76
sleep
apnea 113
cycles 10
disorders 23, 25, 26
slings 101
slowed thinking 14
slurred speech 15, 31-32, 34

small intestine 54
smoking 75, 105, 106, 111-112, 113
cessation medications 111
cessation programs 111
social workers 82, 84
socialization 85
sock donner 100
sodium chloride 107
sound,
hypernasal 32
monotone 32
SP catheter 53
spasticity 37-38, 58
spatial orientation 19
speech 12, 81
and language 27-34
centers 31
pathologist 32, 46, 82, 84, 102
recovery of 27-28
slurred 15, 31-32, 34
therapist 30, 33, 45, 80
therapy evaluation 32-33
sphincter muscles 52
spinal chord 63
split thickness skin graft 67
sprouting 73
stages of swallowing 42-43
standby assist level 81
status epilepticus 62
stimulant laxatives 55
stockings, elastic 61, 101
stool 54
softener 55
strength recovery 36
stretching exercises 38
Stroke Connection 118
stroke research centers 121-122

understanding instructions 37
unmasking 72
upper brain 9
urethra 50
urinary
    devices 58
    tract infections (UTI) 52, 53
urinate 51
urodynamics 51-52
urological evaluation 58
urologists 51, 58, 87
urosepsis 52

V

vasaculitis 111
vascular surgeons 108
ventilation-perfusion scan 60
ventricle 109
vertebrobasilar arteries 11
vertigo 15
videofluoroscopy 45, 46, 48, 49
vision 19, 34, 37, 76, 77
    double 15
    loss 12
    residual 20
    space orientation 9
visual
    feedback 38

field cuts 20, 91
imagery 108
pathways 20
vocal chords 42
voice
    box 27, 42
    tone 27
    volume 27
voiding 51
    pattern 51
voluntary motion 36

W

walker 95
    elevated 83
walking 12, 21-22, 81
    devices 94, 95
warfarin 60, 110, 111
weakness 12, 14, 15, 32, 100
    arm 35
    facial 14
    leg 35
    muscle 36
    on one side 15, 35
    patterns 35
weight change 25
Wernicke's aphasia 31
wheelchairs 96

About the Author

Dr. Kip Burkman graduated from the University of Nebraska College of Medicine in 1984. He completed his residency in physical medicine and rehabilitation at the Rusk Rehabilitation Center in Columbia, Missouri. In 1987 Dr. Burkman joined Immanuel Rehabilitation Center, Omaha, Nebraska, where he serves as Medical Director of Rehabilitation. He is also the Director of the Spinal Cord Injury Rehabilitation Program and the Rehabilitation Center Outpatient Program.

Dr. Burkman is a Fellow of the American Academy of Physical Medicine and Rehabilitation, a Fellow of the American Academy of Disability Evaluating Physicians, and a member of the American Medical Association.

Dr. Burkman also holds a doctor of pharmacy degree from the University of Nebraska College of Pharmacy. He received his undergraduate degree in biology from the University of Nebraska at Omaha in 1976.

Dr. Burkman, his wife Christine, and their two children, Nathan and Alyssa, make their home in Omaha, Nebraska.

Addicus Books
Visit the Addicus Books Web Site:
http://members.aol.com/addicusbks

The Stroke Recovery Book Kip Burkman, MD / 1-886039-30-5	$14.95
Overcoming Postpartum Depression and Anxiety Linda Sebastian, RN, MN, ARNP / 1-886930-34-8	$12.95

The Healing Touch—Keeping the Doctor/Patient
    Relationship Alive Under Managed Care
    David Cram, MD / 1-886039-31-3
	$9.95

Hello, Methuselah! Living to 100 and Beyond George Webster, PhD / 1-886039-25-9	$14.95
The Family Compatibility Test Susan Adams / 1-886039-27-5	$9.95
First Impressions—Tips to Enhance Your Image Joni Craighead / 1-886039-26-7	$14.95
Prescription Drug Abuse—The Hidden Epidemic Rod Colvin / 1-886039-22-4	$14.95
Straight Talk About Breast Cancer Suzanne Braddock, MD / 1-886039-21-6	$9.95

Call Toll Free 1-800-352-2873 (Or order by credit card, personal check or money order)

Please send:

_____ copies of _____ at $ _____ each
(Title of book)

Shipping/Handling $3.00, $1.00 for each additional book.   _____

TOTAL: _____

Name _____

Address _____

City _____ State _____ Zip _____

Phone (____) _____

☐ Visa   ☐ MasterCard   ☐ Am. Express

Credit card number _____ Expiration date _____

Mail to: Addicus Books, P.O. Box 45327, Omaha, NE 68145